"Lisa Campion is a master's master. Her down-to- ⟨...⟩ her breakthrough book. *The Art of Psychic Reiki* ⟨...⟩ many gifted healers of the world come out from hiding and shine the light they were put on Earth to share."

— **Kelly Sullivan Walden,** dream expert and best-selling author of
It's All in Your Dreams

"We are learning that the energetic body is every bit as real as the physical body. This means that a new generation of healers is needed, as we discover more and more about how the release of invisible wounds activates a more powerful, liberated life on every level. I appreciate Lisa Campion's thorough explanation of this work, and how she teaches people to embrace their own healing and their gifts to serve others."

— **Jacob Nordby,** author of *Blessed Are the Weird*

"In her book, *The Art of Psychic Reiki*, Lisa Campion explains in a clear and grounded manner how the system of Reiki goes hand in hand with being a psychic and an empath. This is a wonderful book for anybody who would like to delve deeper into this subject."

— **Frans Stiene,** author of *The Inner Heart of Reiki* and *Reiki Insights*

"*The Art of Psychic Reiki* has made a connection in how learning Reiki can open us even more to ourselves, our recipients, and the world."

— **Rashmi Khilnani,** author of the Reiki master handbook
The Divine Mother Speaks

the
Art
of
Psychic
Reiki

Developing Your Intuitive & Empathic
Abilities *for* Energy Healing

✳

Lisa Campion

REVEAL PRESS

AN IMPRINT OF NEW HARBINGER PUBLICATIONS

Publisher's Note

This publication is designed to provide accurate and authoritative information in regard to the subject matter covered. It is sold with the understanding that the publisher is not engaged in rendering psychological, financial, legal, or other professional services. If expert assistance or counseling is needed, the services of a competent professional should be sought.

Distributed in Canada by Raincoast Books

Copyright © 2018 by Lisa Campion
        Reveal Press
        An imprint of New Harbinger Publications, Inc.
        5674 Shattuck Avenue
        Oakland, CA 94609
        www.newharbinger.com

Cover design by Amy Shoup

Acquired by Jess O'Brien

Edited by Erin Raber

Photograph of Sharon Wilsie by Laura Wilsie

All other artwork by Rosanne Romiglio

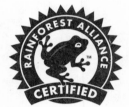

Library of Congress Cataloging-in-Publication Data on file

20   19   18

10   9   8   7   6   5   4   3   2   1   First Printing

Contents

Foreword

Lisa Campion has made a valuable connection between Reiki training, intuition, and psychic ability. Many people who dive into the world of Reiki find themselves opening up to their psychic selves and can feel lost. She has bridged these two worlds in a way that will help those on the path of Reiki to fully step into their potential as healers.

I have been working with Lisa for more than twelve years. She is a highly valued member of my teaching staff at the Rhys Thomas Institute of Energy Medicine. Even before I met her, she was already teaching Reiki and psychic development classes and running a busy healing center. At the Institute of Energy Medicine, we appreciate her compassion for the students and staff. She is a master-level teacher who always finds a way to make challenging or complex spiritual lessons accessible to her students.

Many of the books and classes about Reiki have missed the connection between the practice of Reiki and an increase in intuitive and psychic abilities. This kind of opening is very natural, but it can be shocking for many practitioners. With greater awareness comes greater responsibility. Lisa is a master in this domain and has guided thousands on how to open their intuition in a healthy and safe way.

If you love Reiki and want to take it to the next level of healing, you have picked up the right book. Lisa's compassion and experience as a teacher, healer, psychic, and writer will make this journey deeper into your healing practice a life-changing experience.

—Rhys Thomas
Director of the Rhys Thomas Institute of
Energy Medicine
Author, *Discover Your Purpose*

Why Psychic Reiki?

Reiki is one of the simplest and most intuitive forms of energy healing. It's a gentle, powerful hands-on energy technique from Japan that anyone can learn. (If you aren't yet familiar with the basics of Reiki, you will learn them all in chapter 1.) Learning Reiki can open up our latent sensitivity and our psychic ability. If you are already intuitive and empathic, you may become more so as you go through the levels of Reiki training. Many people have found that when their psychic abilities open up, they feel lost, scared, and confused about what is happening. Sadly, they may even stop practicing Reiki because they are too freaked out about their psychic experiences. This is a terrible loss, because deeply sensitive people are almost always gifted healers.

I believe more than anything that the world needs all the healers it can get. I started practicing as a psychic over thirty years ago, when I was just about twenty years old. I began to weave energy work into my psychic sessions and did all my readings with my clients on a Reiki table. It was a natural combination of modalities for me. I am also a longtime Reiki teacher, and I came to realize that many of my Reiki students needed psychic development as Reiki began to open their sensitivities, so I started teaching them together as Psychic Reiki. Psychic Reiki, which weaves together traditional Reiki training and psychic development, is a perfect pairing. I think it's wonderful that people who study Reiki can expand and develop their psychic natures. All they need is the right training.

My approach to teaching Reiki is experience based and eclectic. All Reiki teachers teach from a different angle, so my hope is that you will benefit from my approach. I'm a big fan of learning from as many teachers as you can, so I honor your previous teachers and hope you learn something from me too. Thank you for making me part of your Reiki journey.

Throughout the book, there are various meditations and exercises to help you explore the principles being described and continue developing your understanding and practice of Reiki. Guided audio for these exercises is available on the publisher's website; visit http://www.newharbinger.com/41214 to find and download the files. (See the very back of this book for more information.)

Introduction

During the two decades that I've been teaching Reiki, I've noticed that my students have tons of natural psychic ability and most are empaths. This makes sense as psychics and empaths tend to be drawn to healing work and have a natural talent for it. Empathy and psychic ability are powerful tools of the healer. Identifying and developing psychic and empathic abilities should be a part of learning Reiki. If you're already psychic and empathic, learning Reiki will open you up deeply and quickly. This can be confusing and frightening if you don't understand what's happening.

Both psychic and healing abilities are by-products of spiritual growth, and Reiki is a powerful spiritual-growth path. Psychic ability expands naturally as we grow spiritually. Yet, there are always bumps along the path that require more integration and growth and Reiki helps immensely with this. Learning Reiki heals us, connects us, and helps us to integrate our healing, psychic, and empathic abilities in a healthy way.

Spiritual Opening, Spiritual Growth

A few years ago, I got a call from my Reiki student Donna. She was in a panic and said, "Ever since your Reiki class, I have been hearing voices at night. I was sure there was someone standing over my bed, praying over me. I could have sworn it was my grandmother, but she died a few years ago!"

I understood why she felt confused and thought she was going crazy. Learning Reiki brought her psychic ability to the forefront very quickly, and she had no idea how to control it or even to understand what was happening to her. Psychic openings can be scary, especially when they happen suddenly. If you already have a lot of latent psychic ability, then learning Reiki can pop open your psychic ability very quickly, which can cause confusion and even panic in people, like it did for Donna.

Many Reiki practitioners begin to have experiences such as the following:

- Seeing colors around people when they are doing Reiki.

- Knowing what the client is feeling physically and emotionally.

- Powerful experiences of the client's energy field, feelings, chakras, and aura. (We'll talk about all these concepts a little later in the book.)

- Sensing the client's blocks, pain, stuck emotions, and other problems.

- Knowing exactly what's happening in a client's body.

- The ability to contact their Reiki guides and angels. (We'll learn about this a bit later in the book as well.)

- Receiving visits from dearly departed souls during a session.

These are all powerful and wonderful experiences, and they can be very helpful to the healing process if you understand what they are. If you don't have the context to understand what it all means, those experiences can be scary and weird.

Donna learned the same processes that I am going to teach you in this book and was able to integrate her psychic ability into her life and also into her Reiki practice. She is now a sought-after practitioner known by her clients for her accurate and helpful psychic insights. When Donna does Reiki she is always aware of her grandmother standing behind her, praying and protecting her. This is comforting for Donna, and she is grateful that she learned what to do when a spirit guide makes contact. It would have been a great loss for her and the world, if she had chosen to deny her psychic and healing gifts out of fear.

Reiki and Spiritual Development

Reiki has a beautiful way of opening the door to a larger world. Many people truly experience energy for the first time after learning the basic level of Reiki. Your hands get very warm when you learn Reiki, and putting your warm hands on other people can help dispel their skepticism. Almost everyone can feel the Reiki energy flowing through them. This feeling of warmth and tingling flow becomes proof that "energy" is real. After that experience, we might then begin to wonder, *What else is real, spiritually speaking?*

Reiki and Healing

Since Reiki heals at physical, emotional, and spiritual levels, you will begin a process of deep self-healing as you learn and practice Reiki. Because Reiki is so accessible, it's a good gateway for anyone exploring what it is to be a healer, especially an energy healer. And, you'll also get some good healing along the way. Part of the miracle of Reiki is that anyone can learn it. You can learn Reiki Level 1 in a few hours and have a very powerful healing modality available to you right away.

Reiki and Intuition

Reiki is an extraordinarily intuitive healing modality. The best Reiki practitioners allow their intuition and their psychic ability to guide the session. The more Reiki you do, the stronger your intuition and psychic ability will be, which in turn makes you a better Reiki practitioner.

Learning and using Reiki is one of the best ways I know of to develop your intuition. The Reiki attunements change your energy field in a way that also supports psychic development. Learning Reiki will help to ground you and strengthen your energy field in many ways that are highly supportive for empaths and sensitives. I recommend that empaths learn Reiki, even if they don't want to do healing work, just to support and strengthen themselves.

Empathy, Psychic Ability, and Intuition

So, what do these words mean—psychic, empath, and intuitive? It sounds like the opening line of a joke: "So, a psychic, an empath, and an intuitive walk into a bar..." Many healers have a package deal of spiritual gifts that all come bundled together. These gifts are intuition, psychic ability, and empathy, the trifecta of healing superpowers.

Empathy

Empaths are emotionally and physically sensitive to others. They are psychic sponges who suck up the emotions and physical feelings of everyone around them. Empaths don't just notice that you are having a feeling; they feel it as if it's *their* feeling. This is a useful quality to have if you are meant to be a healer.

There are two types of empathy. *Physical empathy* is when you put your hands on someone, or are just in physical proximity with them, and you feel in your body what they are feeling in their body. If they have a headache, then you have a headache. *Emotional empathy* happens when you feel someone else's feelings. If you sit next to someone and you're overcome with an emotion, you are probably an emotional empath. (Physical proximity makes it stronger!) This can be challenging until you learn how to manage your empathic response. Empaths need to learn to manage their energy so they don't feel wiped out just by being in the world. If you think about it, empathy is the perfect tool for the healer. It's like a built-in diagnostic tool—your own internal MRI or X-ray machine.

Psychic Ability and Intuition

Psychic ability is our capacity for getting information from outside of our own system. Maybe it's from your grandmother who passed away or your angels. Psychics have an ability to connect with this spirit guidance and receive messages from another realm of reality. Psychic ability can be developed and increased with practice.

Intuition is part of being psychic and consists of *our own inner knowing* and inner wisdom. We have a bad (or good) feeling about

SIGNS THAT YOU MAY BE AN EMPATH

There are characteristics and traits of empaths that distinguish them from other people. If you are an empath, getting the whole picture may help you to make sense of the challenges that you've faced in your life.

- Empaths feel their own feelings very deeply and experience other people's feelings as if they were their own. It's difficult for empaths to discern which of their feelings belong to them and which belong to others.

- Empaths experience anxiety and depression and are prone to addiction.

- Empaths were very sensitive to other people's emotions as children, tuning in to what was going on emotionally in the family.

- Empaths have trouble with boundaries and saying no. They can easily feel "sucked dry" by others.

- Empaths dislike crowds and tend to be introverts. They feel overwhelmed in crowded places, like the movies, the mall, airports, or hospitals.

- Empaths are called to healing, helping, and service work.

- Empaths are sensitive to their physical environments and can have food and environmental sensitivities.

- Empaths prefer to be alone, out in nature, or around animals rather than around people. They identify as introverts.

- There are health challenges that empaths are prone to, including autoimmune disorders and fibromyalgia.

- All empaths are psychic and intuitive, and can feel the presence of spirits around them.

- There is a weak, porous quality to an empath's energy field that may cause fatigue, emotional overwhelm, and health problems.

If you have most of these traits, you are an empath!

something. Or, we just *know* something is going to happen. That is what intuition feels like.

Everyone is intuitive, and many of us are psychic. We can grow these gifts if we pay attention to them and act on them. If you have powerful latent gifts, they are part of your life's purpose and it's wise to train them.

Almost all Reiki practitioners report that they receive guidance about what to do with a client during a session. Intuitive "hits" give you access to how your client is feeling, where the emotional and energetic blocks are, and even what is happening in the person's body. It takes practice to learn to decode the information that you are receiving from other people's energy fields, from spirit guides, and from your own internal senses. We'll work on understanding and beginning to develop these abilities in chapter 7.

THE FOUR HARDEST THINGS ABOUT DEVELOPING YOUR PSYCHIC AND INTUITIVE ABILITIES

After teaching thousands of people how to maximize their psychic abilities, I have boiled down the common stumbling blocks that most people encounter. They seem easy in concept but take practice to incorporate into your life.

They are:

- Releasing misconceptions about psychic insight
- Learning to trust your hits
- Paying attention and listening
- Acting on your hits

As we work through the psychic development piece of this book, you'll begin to resolve these dilemmas so that you feel comfortable with all aspects of your psychic, empathic, and intuitive abilities.

What Does It Mean to Be a "Healer"?

There are so many variations on the concept of healing that it's hard to come up with a single simple definition. I happen to have a private practice and work hands-on with my clients, which is what most people think of when they think of a healer.

We can expand the term "healer" to include caregivers and helpers of all kinds. I've known healers who were stay-at-home moms, nurses, massage therapists, hairdressers, waitresses, physicians, therapists, ministers, and teachers, just to name a few. *Healers* have a gift for healing even if they aren't aware of it, don't use it, or aren't in a healing profession.

One of my Reiki students is a brilliant healer and has a strong mother archetype. She has four children and does Reiki on them daily. She also hosts all the children in her neighborhood at her house. Everyone who needs some TLC gets Reiki from her. She also works on her neighbors, loved ones, and even all the neighborhood pets. Her friends call her the "village witch" since everyone goes to her for help. This is her way of being a healer.

Another student of mine is a vice president of human resources in a huge company. Corporate headquarters isn't where you think a healer would work, but Renee is healing there every day. She is reaching people who maybe wouldn't feel comfortable going to a "healer," and yet they are getting just what they need. Renee brought in Reiki practitioners, chair massage, and reflexology to her office for a once-a-month, in-house wellness retreat.

Jean-Paul, another one of my Reiki students, is a lovely man from Barbados whom I met at the nursing home where he worked. While I was volunteering in the nursing home and giving Reiki to the patients, the director saw such a difference in them that she asked me to train the whole staff. Jean-Paul really took to it; his compassionate nature makes it clear that he is a natural healer. He was very pleased to be able to help his patients feel better with a simple touch.

You can see why I have expanded my definition of "healer" to include all these people and more. It's beautiful to see how every person uses their gifts in the unique way that they were meant to. It's also obvious where the dangers lie. Empaths and psychics can become very drained by their gifts if they have not learned to manage their energy. If you're an empath and you feel called to do hospice work or work with the elderly, how might you feel in hospitals or nursing homes? Overwhelmed? Tired and sad?

Untrained empaths feel like raw, open nerves when they're out in public. It's hard to even leave your house and go to the market some days, never mind working in a hospital. It's a terrible catch-22 that all empaths and most psychics are called to bring their gifts into the world, whether they want to or not. We want to help the world and find a way to ease people's suffering. And, yet, that calls us to environments that deeply challenge us.

Empaths and psychics need good basic training and a lot of practice on how to manage their energy—how to ground, protect, and shield ourselves so that we can do the work that we were meant to do. We also need a functional way to process our own emotions.

Who This Book Is For

The *Art of Psychic Reiki* is the first book of its kind that teaches the basic principles of Reiki in conjunction with psychic development and energy-management basics. If you are new to Reiki and want to learn as much about Reiki as you can, this is a great place to start. We will be covering Reiki Level 1 and Level 2 from the ground up, so if you have never studied Reiki before, you will receive an excellent foundational education.

To be a Reiki practitioner, you do need to receive an attunement from a qualified Reiki teacher. This attunement is the process by which the teacher changes your energy field to allow you to access the Reiki energy yourself. If you haven't received an attunement then I invite you to find a practitioner in your area and make an appointment for your first attunement.

The *Art of Psychic Reiki* is perfect for you if you are already practicing basic Level 1 and Level 2 Reiki and have found that Reiki has opened your psychic gifts. I will teach you how to continue to open your psychic ability safely so that you can use your gifts with your clients and in your life.

Since empathic abilities go hand in hand with both Reiki and psychic development, we will learn and practice the fundamentals of managing your energy during a Reiki session so you don't get drained or flooded with other people's emotions and physical symptoms. Sadly, I have seen many talented healers walk away from Reiki because they were never taught how to manage their energy in a way that keeps them grounded and clear. These energy-management techniques are easy to learn and can be used daily to help you ground, clear your energy field, and stay shielded in any situation. These simple but powerful energy-management techniques will also have a profound impact on your daily life and your work as a healer.

What Else You Will Learn

Learning basic energy anatomy is key to helping you understand and manage your energy as you work with other people's energy. We will explore the basics of the *chakras* (the body's energy centers) and the *aura* (the energy field surrounding people and other beings).

In chapter 4, there is material for supersensitive empaths, too. As I have mentioned, many empaths are drawn to Reiki, and learning it can help us fully understand our empathic natures. It can be very painful to be an empath until we learn how to manage this gift.

With Reiki Level 1, you will learn to do Reiki on your family members and friends, on yourself, and even on your pets. I love to teach the hand positions to use with a person sitting in a chair, since many people don't have access to a Reiki table. I call this "Kitchen Table Reiki," and I have done many healings for people at my own kitchen table.

Here, we will explore how to do Reiki with children, teens, and animals. This is where you will learn the practical application of Reiki so that you can take it out of theory and use it in all kinds of situations in your everyday life. We will also delve into how to deepen your psychic abilities since the goal of this work is to help you access your psychic insight when you need it. It's also important to learn how to turn off your psychic insight when it's not needed so that you are in control of this gift. This chapter is packed full of practical, concrete exercises to deepen your psychic ability that anyone can do.

My hope is that you take advantage of the psychic opening that Reiki training so often brings so that you can use this guidance in every aspect of your life. Your life will be enriched by allowing and following your guidance, since that guidance comes not only from your spirit guides but is also the voice of your own soul. I know that many people are drawn to practicing Reiki because they are seeking a more soulful life and love the spiritual opening that comes with studying Reiki.

Reiki Level 2, which requires a separate Level 2 attunement from a Reiki teacher, is called the Practitioner's Level. Chapter 6 of the book will help you transition from working on your friends and family into a Reiki practice. At this level you can begin to charge money for your Reiki sessions and see paying clients. With Reiki Level 2, you will learn three of the Reiki symbols and how to use them in your healings, as well as the hand positions for someone lying on a Reiki table. We'll also cover more advanced healing practices, such as how to help your client through an emotional release. We want our clients to feel comfortable in expressing their emotions, and yet I find many Reiki practitioners shy away from this crucial part of the healing since they don't feel confident in helping someone with a deep emotional release. One of the most useful skills you'll learn in Reiki Level 2 is long-distance healing. It's wonderful to be able to send Reiki to anyone who needs it, just like a prayer.

In chapter 6, we will also work on deepening and expanding your psychic abilities and will introduce you to the concept of personal Reiki guides. Your guides are benevolent and helpful spiritual healers, and they are already working with you whether you know it or not! Most people find this the most enjoyable and interesting part of the Psychic Reiki program. And, some people can get nervous about it. We will help you work through any anxiety you feel about the topic and connect you to your own unique guides.

Reiki Level 3 is the called the Master Level, which also requires an attunement. At this level, practitioners learn the Master Symbols and how to give Reiki attunements to other people, which is one of the most wonderful things you can do in Reiki! This level of Reiki is beyond the scope of this book, but I hope you will be inspired by your practice and move on to this deeper level of healing.

CHAPTER 1

Reiki Fundamentals

In this chapter, I am going to introduce you to some of the fundamentals of Reiki healing. We need to have this baseline knowledge to help us understand what Reiki is and how it works to heal us. It's beneficial to understand the fundamental principles, such as where Reiki came from and how it works to bring about healing. You'll be introduced to the Reiki Tenets, which provide a solid and beautiful philosophy from the founder of Reiki. We will explore the three levels of Reiki, address how to find a good Reiki teacher near you, and begin the conversation about Reiki's power to change lives in a very tangible way.

Many years ago, I had a friend whose five-year-old boy was in the hospital with leukemia. I went to visit her to help her and her son. I gave her the Reiki Level 1 attunement and taught her some easy hand positions for herself and her son. I spent maybe an hour doing it, and then I left.

When I returned a few days later, she had become a Reiki machine! She was doing Reiki on her son, the kid in the bed next to her son, the parents of that kid, and all the nurses who came through. In the quiet moments of the night, she would do Reiki on herself and pray.

Her son got better and is a handsome and healthy young man now. I have no doubt that Reiki helped her get through that time. It gave her something to do, it helped her feel empowered in a tough situation, and, of course, the energy of Reiki helped everyone receive some healing, too. *That* is the miracle of Reiki.

My friend didn't have time to spend three years in energy medicine school; she needed something she could do right then and right there. She told me that she loved how hot her hands got, because then she knew it was working. No one could deny it, not even her skeptical husband, who also felt better after her Reiki treatments. She said, "I didn't even know what I was doing. I just slapped my hands on people wherever I could, and then I would feel the heat pouring out of me, and everyone got very relaxed and happy after that."

Because Reiki is so intuitive, she was able to loosen up and follow her intuition. Now she's a Reiki Master and works in a hospital volunteering Reiki sessions with patients. She's an angel in that hospital, where she also teaches Reiki to the staff. She's just spreading the Reiki love around!

What Is Reiki?

Reiki (pronounced RAY-key) is a gentle, powerful hands-on technique that uses the Universal Life Force energy around us to heal the body, mind, emotions, and spirit. Reiki is about learning to flow Universal Life Force energy through your body and directing it to another person. It reduces stress, promotes relaxation, and allows everyone to tap into unlimited life-force energy to improve health and enhance the quality of life.

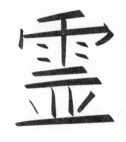

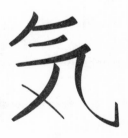

The word "Reiki" derives from two Japanese characters, or *kanji*. *Rei* is the kanji for "spirit," and *ki* means "life-force energy." Together, *Reiki* means "spirit energy" and is generally defined as healing with universal life-force energy.

Reiki can be done on a person lying on a massage table or sitting in a chair. The person receiving Reiki does not get undressed. The Reiki practitioner puts their hands on the client and leaves their hands in one area for a few minutes before moving on to the next area. The recipient might feel heat, a glowing energy, a tingling sensation, or nothing at all. It works regardless of whether you feel the energy or not. Reiki can also be done with the hands off the body, not touching the client at all.

Reiki is a healing modality, but it's also much more. It's a complete system of personal and spiritual growth that includes:

- Meditation practices

- Living by the five Reiki Tenets (guidelines for living a good life)

- Initiations called attunements

- Hands-on healing practices, including self-healing

We will study all these aspects of Reiki throughout the course of this book.

Reiki and Self-Healing

Of all the miracles of Reiki, self-healing is the biggest. Once you know Reiki, you can take advantage of it and do self-healing treatments every day. Self-healing is simple, and it will have a huge impact on your life and ability to do Reiki.

You can do self-healing when you're falling asleep in bed, or even while you're watching TV. Sometimes I do Reiki on myself with one hand while I'm driving. I will take any chance I get to sit quietly and practice self-care. It's just so easy to put my hands on myself and flow a little love my own way.

I also do Reiki on myself when I'm meditating, and I find that it deepens my meditations considerably. It's a beautiful form of self-love, since the nature of Reiki is unconditional love. If you're wondering what you can do to love yourself more, start with some Reiki, just for you. People use Reiki self-healing techniques for things like depression, anxiety, and insomnia. It's also wonderful for fatigue and chronic pain. Reiki can be the first thing in your toolkit that you reach for when you don't feel well.

Is Reiki a Religion?

Reiki is *not* a religion. Reiki is compatible with whatever religious or spiritual beliefs you already have. Reiki is a healing technique, just like yoga, massage, or acupuncture. Sadly, there are some religions that take a negative view of Reiki, including the Catholic Church. I'm not sure why the Church made the decision that Reiki is bad, but it can only come from not understanding the true nature of Reiki.

What Can Reiki Do?

Reiki heals on many levels—the physical, mental, emotional, and spiritual. Because Reiki can be done off the body, it's good for people who are in too much pain to be touched, such as cancer patients and people suffering from rheumatoid arthritis or fibromyalgia.

Reiki is also used for stress reduction and relaxation, which makes it a very popular modality in spa settings. In my private practice, I receive many requests for help with depression and anxiety. I have found Reiki very effective in helping people handle emotional distress. In hospitals, it is used for pre- and postsurgery conditions and pain management with great effect.

There are many other homegrown uses for Reiki, too. You might use it on your kids or other loved ones when they get hurt or feel sick, or when you have a friend crying over a broken heart. When you're tired and cranky, and you don't want to go to work, Reiki yourself!

Who Can Learn Reiki?

The most amazing thing about Reiki is that it takes no special training or prior knowledge. Anyone can learn Reiki in a matter of a few hours and walk away with a powerful, life-changing healing ability. You need no prior experience, nor do you have to have any special talents as a healer. The ability to use Reiki is transferred to the student by the teacher through a technique called an attunement. It's necessary to receive the attunement from a Reiki teacher. If you want to receive an attunement from me, please contact me via my website, or find a teacher near you.

The attunement permanently changes your energy field in a way that lets Reiki flow through you. The attunement process opens the heart, crown, and palm energy centers and creates a special link between the student and the universal Reiki source. The teacher then explains and demonstrates its use. After the attunement, the student simply places his or her hands on someone with the intention of healing and the Reiki energies will automatically flow through the practitioner to the recipient.

The Rise and Spread of Reiki

A Japanese man, Mikao Usui, created Reiki around 1922. Usui Sensei was a martial artist and a spiritual seeker. ("Sensei" is an honorific Japanese title meaning teacher and is the respectful way to refer to instructors.) According to Bronwen and Frans Stiene (2008), he practiced a form of Zen Buddhism called Tendai that included meditation, chanting, chi-moving exercises, and hands-on healing. It's important to understand that Usui Sensei didn't set out to create a hands-on healing modality. He was deeply interested in a system of spiritual practices and philosophy designed to bring his students to enlightenment. Some people think that Usui Sensei rediscovered an ancient art of healing, the same method that Jesus and Buddha used to heal, but according to the Stienes, Usui Sensei studied and taught a deeper form of spiritual practice and discovered the ability to do hands-on healing as part of that process.

Hands-on healing ability, as well as psychic ability, is a by-product of spiritual growth, which is true regardless of what system you are using. Mystics off all kinds, whether they were the Christian mystics, Tibetan lamas, gurus from India, or Japanese Buddhists, have all come across the same spiritual truth, that this kind of spiritual practice leads to healing and psychic abilities. Reiki healing is the birthright of all humans. It's a potential everyone has inside of them, waiting to be awakened and activated by the Reiki attunement.

As Reiki came to America, it lost much of its mystical foundations. Even though modern Westerners focus mainly on the hands-on healing aspect of Reiki, the process will still create a path to spiritual and personal growth despite the newfangled way of practicing it. I believe that is why people are drawn to Reiki whether they know it or not. However, it is still very important for Reiki practitioners to honor the teachers who came before and thank them for their service to the world and to Reiki. Honoring your teachers is a strong part of the Reiki tradition.

This following set of principles is posted on the wall of Usui Sensei's school, and it sums up his philosophy very nicely.

The Ethical Principles of Reiki by Usui Sensei

Just for today do not worry.

Just for today do not anger.

Honor your parents, teachers and elders.

Earn your living honestly.

Show gratitude to everything.

As more nurses and physicians learn Reiki, it is gaining more acceptance in places like hospitals and nursing homes. Research shows the positive impact Reiki has in hospitals, and many now offer Reiki in alternative medicine units. These hospitals have whole teams of Reiki practitioners that are available to you during your hospital stay.

The optimal recipe for healing includes the best that Western medicine offers, along with the best of the alternative therapies that are available. It's great that we get to have both! In recent years, there have been some very good scientific studies about the effectiveness of Reiki and other energy medicine techniques on healing. Scientists are learning how to measure and prove the existence of the human energy field. Reiki has been proven to help in both pre- and postsurgery recovery and to reduce the negative side effects of chemotherapy in cancer patients. Let's hope that with continued research, Reiki will become more and more accepted in hospitals everywhere.

FINDING A TEACHER

When looking up the word Reiki online, it came up with at least 250 different styles of the healing modality. Reiki has naturally evolved and spread, much like how yoga has. When you're looking for a Reiki teacher, finding someone that resonates with you is more important than the style or lineage.

You might consider things like:

- Location and cost

- Program length/time commitment

- Teacher's experience (Check their testimonials and references or get a word-of-mouth referral.)

- Specialization (If you have a specific interest in Reiki, such as Reiki for animals and children or hospital work, it's very likely that you can find a teacher who specializes in that.)

Don't hesitate to speak to the instructor before you sign up with them. Ask questions to see if it's a good fit for you. Good luck finding a teacher! Your intuition will guide you to the right one for you.

The Three Levels of Reiki

There are three levels of Reiki, which are always taught in progression. Some teachers have strict rules about how much time you should spend practicing between levels, but I feel that every person instinctively knows how fast they should go.

I tend to trust the inner wisdom and knowing of my students to tell them how quickly they should progress. Some people feel the need to move quickly and will study all three levels one right after the other. Others take their time. Some people only take Reiki Level 1 and feel no desire to go further, while others go all the way.

However, it's beneficial to give your system a little bit of time between each level to adjust to the changes in your vibration.

In this book, I will teach you the fundamentals of Psychic Reiki: Level 1 and Level 2. Level 3 Reiki is very advanced, and though a book can be an important part of learning it, by the time you are embarking on Level 3 you should have a teacher.

Reiki Level 1: Physical Healing, Self-Healing, and Energy Management

Once you're attuned to Level 1, you'll have Reiki in your hands all the time, so everything you touch will get Reiki automatically. When you're *focused* on giving Reiki, it becomes more powerful. The most powerful aspect of Reiki Level 1 is learning to do self-healing, The Reiki Level 1 attunement can provoke a very mild detox effect in the body. Sometimes hidden physical issues will emerge to be diagnosed and then healed, which makes self-healing even more important.

At Level 1, I'll teach hand positions for people sitting in a chair, which is very useful to know. I'll also teach basic energy management, such as grounding, clearing, and shielding/psychic protection techniques. This helps you learn to work with people without picking up their residual energy.

At Reiki Level 1, we learn and experience the following:

- Receive the Reiki Level 1 attunement (find a teacher near you for this)

- Learn self-healing techniques

- Focus on healing on the physical level

- Learn energy-management techniques for sensitives

- Use basic hands positions for someone sitting in a chair

Reiki Level 2: Emotional and Mental Healing, Working with Others, and Psychic Development

At Level 2, you'll learn three of the Reiki symbols and how to do long-distance healing. At Level 2, you may practice Reiki on people outside the circle of your family and friends. Many people who work hands-on with other people (for example, nurses, massage therapists, body workers, physical therapists, hairdressers, nail technicians, and so forth) should study to Level 2 if possible.

Often, there's a noticeable increase in psychic awareness after a Level 2 attunement, so I teach basic psychic development at this level. Learning to connect with your Reiki guides is one of the most fun and satisfying aspects of this level.

Level 2 provides an opportunity for deep emotional healing. If there are submerged or denied emotional issues, they will gently emerge to be healed and cleared within a few months of a Reiki Level 2 attunement.

At Reiki Level 2, we learn and experience the following:

- Receive the Reiki Level 2 attunement (Find a teacher near you for this.)

- Learn Reiki Level 2 symbols for physical healing, emotional healing, and mental healing

- Learn long-distance Reiki healing techniques

- Cultivate our psychic insight and intuition

- Connect with our Reiki guides and develop basic psychic skills

- Learn Reiki hand positions for someone on a table

Reiki Fills Us First

As practitioners, Reiki energy flows into the tops of our heads and down the spine. Some of it flows down the legs into the ground, giving us a firm connection to the earth, so it's very grounding. Then the energy flows up the front of the body and into our hearts, down the arms, coming out the palms of the hands, and flowing into our recipient.

Because Reiki flows like this, it fills us first, restoring our energy before we start working on someone else. You may notice that you feel more energized and peaceful after you do a Reiki session. You can think of it as filling your own cup until that cup runs over. If you're doing work like massage therapy, adding Reiki will increase your stamina considerably.

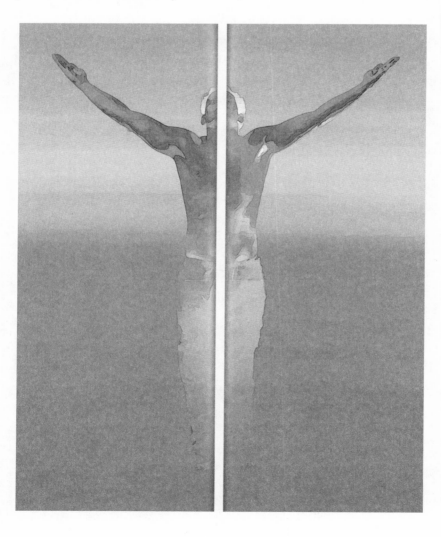

Reiki Heals Through Love and Life-Force Energy

It's an old adage that love heals, but it's true. Reiki is love in a frequency that we can all access. Reiki is good at healing wounds around love, so it works well for grief (loss) and shame (self-hatred). If you practice Reiki on yourself, you're much more likely to have a loving relationship with yourself!

Reiki also brings Universal Life Force energy to areas in your body that need it. We call this energy *ki* or *chi*. This means increased circulation and oxygenation to places that need it. Body tissues begin to break down when there's not enough blood flowing freely; our blood brings nutrients and oxygen to our bodily systems and removes waste products from the cells.

Reiki also works by releasing stuck and stagnant emotions from body tissues and from our energetic system. When we don't allow ourselves to express our feelings, they can get packed away in the cells of the body. This is *always* bad for us. Nerve cells and tissues hold unresolved trauma, and muscle, organ, and fat tissues hold unexpressed emotions.

These pent-up emotions create blocks in the flow of *chi* through the body and are a big source of long-term health issues. For example, let's say you're a person who never lets yourself cry. You shut down your heart and soldier on, holding all your grief and pain inside. You even hold your breath to shut down emotions. This shuts down the heart energy center over and over again. After twenty or thirty years of doing this, the actual muscle and tissue of your heart weakens and chronic physical problems begin to develop.

Reiki helps release that stuck emotional energy from wherever you're holding it. Sometimes people will have an emotional release while receiving Reiki. They may cry, laugh, or feel angry. This is very healing! If your recipients should have an emotional release (for example, they start crying), just be as supportive as you can. Reiki their heart, hold their hand, and let them talk about anything that comes up. Comfort them as best you can; support them as if they were a friend that came to cry on your shoulder.

Reiki also heals by relaxing the recipient. When we relax, the body's natural healing capabilities kick in. There have been many scientific studies that prove that stress is a huge killer. Anything we can do to relax and de-stress adds to our sense of well-being.

Reiki Goes Where It's Needed

Reiki is foolproof, because Reiki *knows* where to go. The energy flows to the spot people need it to, without either you or them having to think about it. When you put a sponge under running water, the water flows to every area of the sponge that is dry. The sponge and the water don't *try* to make this happen, it just does. It's the same thing with Reiki. The people receiving the Reiki *pull* the Reiki to the place they need it most, just like the dry sponge pulls the water to the dry spot.

Reiki energy flows like water through our systems. This allows it to fill in the spots that really need it. When we're doing Reiki, we trust in the innate wisdom of our recipient's system, which will pull the Reiki where it needs to go.

The Takeaway

I hope you now have a better understanding about the fundamentals of Reiki. It's important to get some basic information, such as where Reiki came from, how it's being used in the world now, and how it works. You learned about how Reiki helps us heal us by:

- Vibrating at the frequency of unconditional love

- Connecting us with Universal Life Force energy

- Bringing life-force energy to tissues in the body that lack good circulation and energy

- Releasing stuck and unexpressed emotions from the body tissues

- Invoking relaxation to kick in the body's natural healing capabilities

In the next chapter, you are going to learn more about how psychic abilities work. It's a lot easier than you might think, especially if you are willing to let go of some common misconceptions that people have about what being psychic is like. Let's jump into the reality of your psychic gifts. You will be amazed by how psychic you already are.

CHAPTER 2

Understanding and Awakening Your Psychic Gifts

Who is psychic? As it turns out—everyone! Being psychic is innate in humans; it's an ability that evolved with us as a species. It's *so* natural, that you're probably already way more psychic than you think you are!

Most people have a dramatic idea of what being psychic is based on media portrayals of psychics. Real psychic hits are so much more subtle, useful, and part of everyday life. Here are some examples of everyday psychic experiences. Pay attention to which of these might feel familiar to you.

- Have you ever known something was going to happen before it did? This *inner knowing* is often felt in the belly, as a gut feeling. Or, you might be able to assess people very quickly. If you are naturally a great judge of character, it means you are using your intuition to energetically read people for their character and their intentions.

- Do you sometimes see something out of the corner of your eye, and when you turn your head, there is nothing there? This is an indication of *visual psychic skills*. Visual psychics also dream frequently and intensely. If you have ever had a dream that came true, or have been visited in your dreams by a relative who has passed over, then you may well have this gift.

- Empaths are very tuned to the *emotional channels* and their strongest psychic sense is their feelings. "I have a bad [or good] feeling about this..." is something an empath will say. These feelings can extend to feeling creeped out in someone's house, or having a funky feeling about a person. Empaths receive very accurate psychic information through their emotional channels and need to learn to trust them.

- Do you hear things when nothing or no one is there? People with strong *auditory psychic skills* might hear their name called out loud when no one is there, or "hear" a little voice in their head that is giving them good advice. It can be very simple and practical: *Don't forget your brief-case!* Or, it can be quite strong and loud: *Watch out! Danger ahead!*

If you have had *any* of these experiences, then you have had a psychic experience. In this chapter, we are going to learn how to begin to weave your psychic ability into your Reiki practice and your daily life. We need to start with letting go of some misconceptions that people have about being psychic and discover the four big mistakes you can make that shut down your psychic ability. We will also explore the psychic senses to be able to understand from which channels your psychic information is coming to you.

Intuition vs. Psychic Insight

Intuition and psychic insight are connected, but they are not the same thing. *Intuition* is our own innate wisdom. It's information coming from within ourselves: our body wisdom, our feelings and emotions, and our inner knowing. If we're tuned in to it, it works like a powerful inner navigation system that guides us through life. Intuition has three major components:

- Your body wisdom and truth. Your body never lies and always knows what's real. *I always feel sick (or good) when they're around.*

- Your emotions and feelings, and your empathy. *I have a good [or bad] feeling about that.*

- Your gut knowing that you feel in your belly. *I don't know why I know, I just know.*

It's powerful when all three elements of your intuition agree, and, luckily, they usually do. Intuition tells us to go in the direction our soul is calling us to, and away from the wrong path. It comes as pressures, nudges, urges, desires, and aversions. Intuition is guidance from your higher self. I think of the higher self as an interface that our own soul uses to speak to us. It's the part of us that stands in between the soul and the personality as an intermediary. It's because intuition gives you direct access to your own soul that it is so important and powerful.

Psychic information comes from *outside* our own system. This is information delivered to us from our guides. I use the term *guides* to denote all the helpful, benevolent spiritual beings who work with us. We all have a team of guides—angels, spiritual teachers, and loved ones who have passed over—who want to help us.

Psychic insight is our ability to clearly access the information our guides give us, and this insight comes from outside our own system. Psychic information is harder to access than intuitive information, so it takes more training. We need to learn to decode the messages we get from our guides, since they often speak in the language of symbols. It takes training to activate and polish our psychic insight, but it's so worth doing.

Misconceptions About Psychic Ability

Psychic ability and intuitive ability are a lot more accessible than most people think. It's expectations, misconceptions, and our ego that make it hard to receive information from spiritual sources. The most common misconception is that being psychic is difficult, and only special people can do it. Another common misconception is that it only counts if it's a dramatic vision, like those TV psychics have.

We're used to seeing psychic ability as a phenomenon portrayed in the media. We see the TV psychic overcome with a powerful vision. It's so disturbing and upsetting that the psychic flops down on the floor, twitching and overcome with emotion. They are haunted and obsessed by what they see, and what they see often involves violent crimes.

When people compare their experience to those stories, they think they must not be psychic because it's not like that. Often, when people first experience an authentic psychic connection, they'll say, "Is *that* all it is? That was way too easy!" or "I've been hearing that voice in my head my whole life! I just thought it was my imagination!" Here are some misconceptions to drop before you go further on this path:

- Only special people are psychic.

- It only counts if it's a vision. (Truthfully, all the other psychic senses are more reliable and much more common, as we'll see.)

- A psychic experience comes with a lot of fanfare and is a big deal.

- It's really hard and you have to try, try, and try!

- Being psychic is not a normal, everyday part of life.

- Only crazy people are psychic; therefore, all psychics are crazy.

Psychic experiences are woven into your daily life in a very natural and organic way. Sometimes, we have a very pronounced, peak psychic experience, but most of the time it's a very subtle and natural experience. Developing your psychic ability is like developing any other natural ability; you need to learn to trust yourself, pay attention, and practice taking action.

Learning to Trust Yourself

I've seen many people get a perfectly good psychic hit and dismiss it as nothing. Often this comes down to a powerful argument between the mind and the heart. The thinking mind is the least psychic organ we have. It's all about logic and analysis. Can you remember a time when you had an intuitive hit, but your mind talked you out of it? It probably looked something like this:

Your Intuition: *Pssst! Hey! I really don't like that person. They are yucky and creepy—run away, quick!*

Your Mind: *What are you talking about? I'm sure that's a perfectly nice person! Don't be silly!*

Your Intuition: *Ugh. Nope. No way. Don't trust that person at all.*

Your Mind: *That's ridiculous! Look around! Everyone else likes this person. You're just imagining it all. Again! I am not listening to you, so shut up!*

Your Intuition: *Okay, if you say so! But, I'm going to say, "I told you so!" when things go bad.*

You know how this plays out, right? Your intuition will have been right about that person the whole time. We need to quiet and calm our minds and trust that our first gut instincts and impressions are almost always right.

Paying Attention and Listening

Ninety percent of being a good psychic is about paying attention to what is happening in you and around you all the time. It sounds simple, but it can be difficult to practice. It means changing the bad habits that you have, like zoning out or disconnecting from yourself.

The following behaviors are ways to pay attention and listen:

- Tune in to your body at all times. Your body is the best psychic barometer you have.

- Notice your feelings all the time.

- Be open to receive what your guides and your own intuition are saying. Listen to the inner voices.

- Be aware of the world around you and look for signs and omens.

- Listen to how your subconscious and intuitive parts talk to you, such as through your dreams, your feelings, and your hunches.

Once you start paying attention, you'll realize that you're getting many hits all day long. But, you'll miss all of them if you're constantly tuned out. It takes a lot of practice to change the habit of being tuned out. We'll start by learning and practicing grounding techniques, which we'll cover in chapter 3.

Grounding and other energy-management techniques also help us avoid being swamped by too much psychic information. Learning to master your psychic skills allows you to regulate the flow of information, so that your psychic insight is off when you want it off, like when you are in the supermarket, but on when you want it on, like when you are in a Reiki session. This is one of the most important parts of psychic development, since being *on* all the time isn't very pleasant. Many people struggle with being able to turn off their gifts when they really need to.

Acting On Your Hits

If you get a hit but don't act on it, you're showing that you're not serious about your guidance. This is the number one mistake that most people make, and it will turn *off* your psychic insight and intuition. This doesn't mean that you must act on every single hit or follow through on the more outlandish ones. But, it does mean that you should honor your intuition and your insight by giving them a high priority in your life.

A hit could be something as small as *Something is wrong at home, you better check in,* or as big as *Time to get divorced right now!* You can see why we so often don't listen! A lot of the time, our big hits move us out of our comfort zones. Your own soul (which is always your best guide) and your spiritual guides feel a lot of compassion for your pain and fear of change, but they aren't interested in keeping you small or in your comfort zone.

Not too long ago, I started getting a strong message
guides every time I did my evening meditation: *Quit eating sugar...*
would roll my inner eye and shrug it off. I didn't want to quit eating
sugar! It's hard to quit, and I like my chocolate. This went on for
almost a year, with the volume going up on the message almost every
day.

One day, my guides gave me a pretty stern talking to. If I wouldn't
listen to the simple stuff, how was I going to handle big messages and
big changes? About a week after that, I went to my regular yearly
health exam and guess what? My blood sugar was high. My doctor
looked me in the eye and said, "You need to quit eating sugar!"

When we use our psychic insight and intuition correctly, they
propel us forward on our spiritual path despite the fear and trepida-
tion our personalities feel, and that is always good for us in the long
run. Honoring your hits by acting on them strengthens your psychic
muscle and gives you more intense and stronger hits. Ignoring them
makes your psychic muscle atrophy.

Developing Your Psychic Abilities Safely

When we work on psychic development, it's very important that we
work safely. If you do it properly, you'll be fine. If you don't, you could
open yourself up to a host of bad situations. My best analogy is that
psychic development is a lot like street smarts: If you're street savvy,
you can walk around in a big city anywhere on the planet and be
safe, but if you aren't, you can get into a lot of hot water. Avoid
trouble by following these guidelines:

- Do your grounding, clearing, and shielding/psychic protection practices every day. (We will cover these fundamentals later in the book.)

- Don't undertake psychic development unless you are
  already in good mental health. You need a firm foundation of mental health, since psychic development can
  throw you further off balance if you're already on shaky
  ground.

- Don't mix psychic development with drug or alcohol use.

- Stay away from unsafe practices like the Ouija board. Spirit boards, like the Ouija board, seem harmless enough. They are in the games sections at toy stores after all! However, they open a portal to a darker place that most of us don't want to deal with. It's a doorway to the lower astral plane, and no good can come from visiting that place. It's the psychic equivalent of a bad neighborhood. People who "play" with a spirit board can open a permanent portal to this place in their house. The Ouija board can initiate some powerful and very negative hauntings.

- Don't look for trouble. (In other words, don't take the Ouija board to the abandoned mental hospital on Halloween while doing a lot of drugs.)

- Don't do ghost hunting unless you get excellent training.

- Don't play around with dark practices just to see if anything happens.

- Don't share your psychic hits with people unless they ask for it. It's rude to blurt out your hits to unsuspecting people; it's a violation of their privacy.

- Always practice in an ethical way and respect the power of your word as a psychic and a healer.

Some people get into trouble because they don't really believe in the spiritual world. Most of the things that you see on paranormal TV shows are highly dangerous for amateurs. When you don't believe in the spiritual world, it seems like all fun and games to poke around in it, just to see what happens. Don't. It's like not believing in sharks and then chumming the water and jumping in, just to see if sharks are real. If you use common sense, are respectful, and apply your street smarts, psychic development is perfectly safe.

❀ *Samira's Story* ❀
Reclaiming Psychic Gifts

Samira had been very psychic as a child, with the complete package of psychic skills. She could see things, hear things, and feel everything, too. She was gifted at sensing the future before it happened. When she was little, her very accurate predictions about deaths and pregnancies upset her family, and she was punished for them.

Samira was visited by spirits every night. They kept her awake by talking to her. She remembers her mother praying over her so it would stop happening. When she was seven years old, she asked God to take her gifts away so she could be "normal." The occurrences eventually became less dramatic, and she stopped talking about them. Everyone in her family was relieved. Her psychic experiences moved to her dreams, and she had very restless sleep with a lot of nightmares and insomnia, even as a child. She was visited by spirits of the dead every night in her dreams and had strong premonitory dreams.

As an adult, Samira trained as a therapist and was drawn to the healing arts. She practiced yoga and did regular meditation, both of which increased her psychic ability. When she learned Reiki, she was no longer able to contain her psychic ability. She found that she was ready to stop squashing it. It had become clear to her then, in her late thirties, that the "gift" was not really a curse, but a real gift that she was meant to use in her healing work. As she took my psychic development classes, she blossomed and expanded into her impressive psychic gifts. She became a highly sought-after healer who has combined her psychotherapy with Reiki and deeply powerful intuitive work.

The Psychic Senses

Our psychic senses are an extension of our physical senses. ESP (extrasensory perception) is a very accurate description of how we experience our psychic ability. Here's a quick breakdown of the psychic senses. As you read them, you'll probably be able to see which ones are naturally strongest in you. Don't forget, it's totally possible to have all these psychic gifts or any combination of them.

The Visual Psychic Sense (Clairvoyance)

This is the psychic sense that most people really want, however, it's actually rare. It is the most painful and difficult ability to have, because visual psychics often feel like they're crazy. Historically, visual psychics have been the most persecuted and feared. Not too long ago, if you had this gift, you might have been thrown into a mental hospital for seeing angels, fairies, or your dead relatives. Since this skill is usually more intense when we're children, being a visual psychic can make for a rocky, frightening, and disturbing childhood.

I'm a visual psychic and spent most of my childhood hiding this from other people and trying to act "normal" in public. I spent the first twenty years of my life trying to figure out how to turn it off. I was tuned in to some pretty scary things. Ghosts, shadow spirits, and the creepy energy of other people's families and houses were a daily experience for me. I also saw wonderful things, like angels and earth spirits, but a lot of times I didn't know what they were.

While it has a sexy reputation, visual psychic ability is the most unreliable and hard to interpret. My classes are full of people trying to develop and strengthen their psychic abilities, except for that one visual psychic who's freaked out and trying to turn it off! Though it's challenging, clairvoyance is an amazing ability to have. It does require more training than the other psychic skills, but a well-trained visual psychic is a very powerful healer. Here are some ways visual psychic ability shows up:

- You see something out of the corner of your eye, and when you turn your head there is nothing there. Our peripheral vision is the part of our optics that is best tuned to seeing psychic phenomena.

- Most visual psychics will be able to see energy around people, especially when they are doing Reiki. You might see colors, light, or energy moving.

- Visual psychics have very detailed and vivid dreams that they remember upon waking.

- Visual psychics have vibrant imaginations and the ability to visualize things is easy.

Sometimes it can be difficult to tell the difference between a visual psychic hit and your imagination. Your imagination responds easily to your will. If I tell you to imagine a pink elephant, you can. A hit comes on its own. If you try for the pink elephant and you see a vision of an angel, that is a real hit. When your visual psychic insight opens, you'll be able to see things when you do Reiki on people. It's a wonderful diagnostic tool for Reiki healers.

SEEING COLORS

Practitioners with strong visual psychic capabilities may begin to see colors around people during a Reiki session. Sometimes we see these colors with our eyes open, but they can also be experienced with the eyes shut. When we "see" with our eyes shut, we are seeing with our inner eye, the psychic eye. In the beginning, it may feel like it's your imagination, but it is the onset of psychic vision.

The colors represent the state of the person you are working on. For example, if you see black, gray, or brown around a certain spot on the body, this is a sign that there is blocked energy or stuck emotions in that part of the body.

One of my Reiki students, Aimee, was practicing on a woman who was going through a divorce and was very sad and grieving. Aimee could see a gray, smokelike energy releasing from this woman's heart. When the smoke cleared, the woman's heart center went back to a nice pink color. This pink color was the woman's heart returning to love.

When Laura first came to my office for a Reiki session, I saw a black cloud all around her. I was not surprised when she told me that she was suffering from severe depression. Over the months we worked together, she began to heal from her trauma. Every time she came in, I would see a change in the color. When she was working through a big piece of anger, I saw her energy field as fiery red. When she was working through grief, she came in looking totally blue, and I realized why we say someone has the "blues."

If you are tapping into the emotions of the Reiki recipient, then the colors might look like this, according to Ted Andrews (2006):

- Red can mean both passion and anger.

- Orange is life-force energy and sexuality.

- Yellow is the will and mental energy (thinking).

- Green is a heart color and the color of healing.

- Pink is love.

- Blue can be either sadness or peacefulness.

- Purple is a very spiritual color and is the color of Reiki.

Often, clients see colors during their Reiki healing, too. Lots of folks see purple when getting a Reiki attunement, which shouldn't be a surprise since purple is the color of Reiki! Sometimes Reiki healers will also see the colors of the energy centers, or chakras, as they are working on their clients. We will learn more about these in chapter 3, but here are the colors associated with them, according to Anodea Judith (2004).

- Red is the earth and root energy center, which represents grounding and our connection to the earth.

- Orange is the color of the navel energy center, which is about passion, sexuality, and pure life-force energy.

- Yellow is the color of the solar-plexus energy center and is about our personal power, will, and self-esteem.

✿ Green is the color of our heart center and is about love, forgiveness, and heart healing.

✿ Blue is the color of the throat energy center and is about communication, speaking, and our creativity.

✿ Indigo is the color of the brow energy center and is about our mind, thinking, and how we see things.

✿ Violet is the color of the crown energy center and is about our connection to the Divine and infinite possibility.

As you gain experience as a Reiki healer, you will begin to see more and more colors on your Reiki recipients, and you will also learn how to tell if what you are seeing is the color of an emotion or one of the energy centers.

The Auditory Psychic Sense (Clairaudience)

The auditory psychic sense is more prevalent than the visual sense. It's also more accurate, and it is generally easier to deal with. If you're clairaudient, you'll hear your guidance as a voice in your head. Most people who hear this initially think it's their own voice, until they learn to distinguish their inner ego-based voice from that of their intuition. The psychic inner voice is a quiet and rather matter-of-fact voice. It sounds different than your ego-based inner voice, which is usually a little uncertain.

Your ego's inner voice may sound like *Gosh, am I doing this right? What was that symbol? I bet I'm not saying it right. I think I should put my hands over here, but I'm not sure.* Your intuitive voice may sound more like *This person is sad and his heart is blocked up, but he's brave and trying not to cry. Put your hands here and don't move until you feel it release. Go!*

Auditory psychics hear things, such as their name being called when there's no one home. If they ask a question, they may hear an inner voice answer. Many people hear a ringing or buzzing in their ears as a sign that their auditory psychic sense is kicking in. Sometimes, that's the cue that your guides want to talk to you. It's like they're ringing you up on the phone.

Auditory psychics tend to be very sensitive to sound in general and often have a deep love of music. As a Reiki practitioner, this is a very handy psychic gift to have. You will notice that you are being guided through the Reiki session as if another voice that is not your own is giving you a set of verbal instructions. Auditory psychics will literally be told how to proceed. You may hear things like *Now move your hand here, this person is angry and it needs to release. Stay here. Okay, now move to this spot.*

The Somatic Psychic Sense

Somatic means in or of the body. Somatic psychics feel things in their bodies; they feel empathy physically. Physical psychic ability is very useful and super reliable. Sadly, it's often overlooked and under-appreciated by those who have it. Your body always knows what's true and what's real, so it's almost impossible to fool. I've learned over the years to trust this psychic sense completely. If my body is reacting, feeling something new, or freaking out, I listen.

To experience the power and accuracy of your somatic psychic sense, start paying attention to what your body tells you about people. Notice if you lean toward or away from someone. Do you want to touch this person, or do you feel repelled? How do you feel when you do touch this person? Pay attention to your chest, heart, and belly.

All psychics have a body signal that lets them know that their guidance is coming in, or that the truth is being spoken. For some people, it's a shiver or some goose bumps. For others, it's a tingle, hot flashes, tummy flips, or hair standing up on the back of the neck. When you feel it, you'll know you're on the right track. Learn your signals and then pay attention!

As a Reiki practitioner, our hands will become more and more sensitive and proprioceptive. My hands are like a barometer that tells me what's happening in a client during a Reiki session. I get a much stronger psychic reading when I have my hands on someone. Since I often do intuitive medical work, touching someone allows me to feel deeply into the body and energy system. If someone really releases during a Reiki session, I'll feel a big swoosh of energy down my own spine, or a change in my breathing. I also feel what my client is feeling in my own body.

Another well-known form of somatic psychic ability is called *psychometry*. Psychics with this ability get their information by touching objects or people. One of my psychic students is gifted in this way. She does very accurate readings for people by holding objects like a wedding ring or a watch. Perhaps not surprisingly, she has an antique shop and a knack for collecting rather haunted and psychically charged objects.

In general, somatic psychics are touch oriented. They often love to be touched themselves, and it's not unusual to find them working in body-oriented jobs, such as massage therapy.

The Empathic Gift

We're going to discuss empaths in depth later, but the short version is that empaths are the psychic sponges of the world. Empaths feel and absorb the energy around them at a much deeper level than any other kind of psychic. This is different than just knowing or having a feeling about something; empaths *feel* other people's emotions and physical issues as if they were their own. It's a very difficult psychic gift to have, and empaths suffer until they learn to manage their gift. But, they make fabulous healers!

If you are an empath, you feel other people's feelings as if they are your feelings and you will experience what others are feeling in your body. These two gifts combined are the perfect diagnostic tool of the healer. Until they learn how to manage their energy, empaths may suffer from anxiety and depression, which is usually someone else's pain and suffering. Because of their extreme sensitivity, empaths avoid crowds and dislike being in busy, public places. Empaths tend to have poor boundaries and difficulty saying no, so they frequently collect needy people around them who tend to drain them.

In chapter 4, we'll discuss how to manage empathic energy so that you can use your gifts fully. You will no longer view being an empath as a crazy curse that you wish you could give back. Instead, you'll be able to fully utilize this amazing gift, the gift of the healer. You will begin to see how empathy, the somatic psychic ability, and the gift of knowing come together to create the intuitive psychic.

The Intuitive Gift

As we have discussed, intuitive psychic ability combines the somatic sense, strong empathy, and gut knowing. It's a beautiful, useful, and accurate set of psychic skills. Basically, if your body, your feelings, and your gut are all in agreement, you can count on the information you are getting as being on point.

Emilio is an intuitive psychic who is an exceptional Reiki healer. He runs a Reiki center in a big city where he holds classes, sees clients, and runs a free Reiki clinic for his neighborhood. He starts getting intuitive information the minute his clients enter his office. He just knows what is going on with them, even if they can't communicate it. Emilio says, "I work with people who live in a culture where it's not cool to confess to having emotions. If you ask how they are feeling, they always say 'fine' even if it's clear that they are not fine." When he starts sessions and puts his hands on his clients, he can feel their emotions and what's happening in their body. He can gently begin to release stuck energy, pain, and emotions. He says, "I have to rely on my intuition, because they would never admit to anything. But, once I get things flowing, they are relieved to talk about it and release it."

Emilio uses his intuition as the guiding force in his own life. "I have faith in my intuition. I know I am guided. I use my intuition constantly through my day, and I swear it's saved my life a few times. I know who to trust and who not to. I know when there is danger, if someone needs help, or there is trouble brewing somewhere. I feel this is part of God's gift to me."

When you get good at it, this ability will feed you continual information about not only your Reiki sessions, but also your life. Since intuition is how our soul speaks to us, it's a form of spiritual practice that will help you live a more soulful life and deeply connect to your life's purpose.

The Gift of Mediumship

Mediums are psychics who have the gift of speaking to the dead. This is a specialized gift that needs its own kind of mentoring and training. Mediums usually exhibit their gifts as children but shut down their abilities when they're not supported. The most powerful mediums have had near-death experiences or other powerful death experiences, like the loss of a loved one. In crossing over and then coming back, they create a strong connection with the other side. This can be a difficult psychic gift to endure without proper training. Being tuned in to the "dead channel" is no fun if you can't turn it off or focus it properly. When a medium is properly trained, he or she has an amazingly healing gift that provides closure for people who really need it. You will know that you have mediumship capacity if the spirits of the dead often surround you. Untrained mediums are "ghost magnets." You may also dream about those who have crossed over, or know when someone is going to die.

❀ *Anna's Story* ❀
Embracing the Gift of Mediumship

Anna had a busy massage therapy practice. She has been able to see the spirits of the dead since she was a child. Anna's family was not afraid of her gift, but they didn't know what to do to support her. She told me that they thought she was making it all up and just had a very active imagination. Her childhood was full of her "imaginary friends."

As Anna went through puberty, her mediumship ability grew much stronger and started to interfere with her life. She had to avoid going out in public if she was tired because she would attract spirits all around her. Anna was a classic "ghost magnet." "Every spirit within a five-mile radius came to visit me at night," she said. And, of course, there was a cemetery just down the road from her.

She studied Reiki, since she wanted to add it to her massage therapy practice, and had loads of natural talent. Learning Reiki activated her mediumship ability even more. "One day, during a massage session, my client's mother suddenly appeared. I didn't want to say what I was seeing and hearing since I didn't want to freak out my client or upset her. What if she thought I was crazy? And, what if I was wrong! So, I said nothing since I didn't know what to do." The next time the same client came for a massage, the spirit of her mother came along with her. Eventually the mother said to Anna, "I am not going to leave you alone until you pass the message along!"

I coached Anna on how to bring this up with her client. It's always important when we get a strong hit to ask permission to share it. Anna's client was very excited to hear the message from her mother. The client cried, Anna cried, and the mother cried, too. Lots of things that needed to be said came through, and then the mother could fully let go and be at peace. And, so was the client.

It was a wonderful experience for Anna, since she began to have more faith in her gifts and she could see how clearly beneficial and healing they were for all concerned. Anna is well known in her town now as the massage therapist medium. She said it was the Reiki and psychic development training that fully brought her gift into the forefront again.

Anna's story is a great example of how this gift of mediumship can blossom into a wonderful healing skill. Mediums can help people heal from the death of a loved one by providing much needed closure for both the living and departed.

Opening to our psychic, intuitive, and empathic abilities is a natural result of studying Reiki. This a marvelous thing, and it's also challenging if we are not ready for it. We are about to start learning about Reiki and develop our psychic abilities.

Practices for Developing and Integrating Your Psychic Ability

When people are looking to strengthen their psychic ability, they are usually searching for ways to ensure that their gifts are operative at their command. There are several ways to develop your psychic abilities through practice and to learn how to turn them on and off. These include automatic writing, divination, and dream interpretation. We'll talk about some of these later in the book. The two most important tools for understanding, accepting, and developing your psychic gifts are keeping a psychic journal and having a spiritual practice.

Keep a Psychic Journal

I recommend getting a dedicated psychic journal that you use to record your hits. This is one of the most powerful tools that you can use for psychic development, since what we pay attention to grows. You will want to record whatever hits you get during the course of the day and during your practice sessions. Maybe it's a gut feeling or a time when your intuition was active.

When you begin to recognize synchronicities, signs, and omens, you can also write those down, too. Your journal can also become a wonderful place to record your dreams, especially if you have trouble remembering them. As we will discuss shortly, writing down any wisps or fragments of dreams is the best way to remember them.

Adding in any psychic experiences you have in your Reiki sessions is especially helpful. They might be colors that you see around people as you're working, or other intuitive hits about how your person is feeling and how you sensed energy moving in the Reiki sessions. As you write down your hits and contemplate them, your psychic journal will become a place where you can analyze the information that you are receiving, since it takes some practice to learn how to interpret our psychic hits. This information often comes through the language of symbols, much like dreams do. I think this is the most difficult aspect of psychic development. You can get the hit, but figuring out what it means takes practice, and your psychic journal is an excellent tool for this.

As you record all your psychic experiences in your journal, you will be amazed at how psychic you really are! It will help you continue to pay attention to all that is happening, which will also help increase your ability.

Maintain a Spiritual Practice

You must commit to a spiritual practice to increase and develop your psychic ability. There is no getting around this. Here's a great analogy: if you want to get in shape, you must work out, and there's no getting around that either! It's that straightforward. Spiritual practice is the psychic's version of working out. We'll only get to a certain level of personal, psychic, and spiritual development before we're stopped dead in our tracks if we don't pick up and keep a spiritual practice. I believe that psychic ability is a by-product of the larger and more important goal of spiritual development, so we need to be committed to growing spiritually through spiritual practice.

What exactly *is* a spiritual practice? It comes in many forms and I don't think it really matters so much *what* you do; it's just important that you pick something and stick with it. It can be a form of sitting meditation, guided meditation, mantra meditation, or prayer. Praying the rosary is a wonderful form of spiritual practice. Other people do better with a body-based spiritual practice like yoga, tai chi, or walking meditation.

If we want to increase our psychic ability, we must make space to get quiet, be receptive, and learn how to listen. All spiritual practices quiet the mind, and clear and open the spiritual energy centers, which is what we need to be able to hear our guides.

I'm a big fan of sitting meditation (sitting still and quieting your mind) and do at least twenty minutes of it every day. Sitting meditation is a difficult one to start with. If you want to do sitting meditation, it's best to take a class and learn a technique that will help you. Many people do better with guided meditations when beginning a practice. If you have an extrabusy mind, mantra meditations and chanting are very effective at quieting busy brains.

Some people really can't and shouldn't do sitting meditation and must stick with a body practice. If you are dissociated to begin with, a body-based practice will benefit you more than sitting meditation. Try a gentle yoga or tai chi. Gym yoga or a very vigorous flow yoga is good exercise but isn't geared toward meditation. Stick with gentle hatha yoga if you're looking for a meditative practice.

Yoga is designed to clear out your energy meridians and physical body so that you can meditate without feeling all blocked and kinked up. We tend to get the balance backward: fifty minutes of yoga and only five minutes or so of meditation at the very end. Ideally, we should do twenty minutes of yoga to clear our energy fields, and then twenty to thirty minutes of meditation afterward.

Empaths do particularity well with a "walk-the-dog" kind of meditation, especially if they can walk in the woods. Being out in nature clears the energy field naturally and easily, and it calms and clears the whole system.

When you're first starting a spiritual practice, aim for five times a week, ten to fifteen minutes at a time, and grow it from there if you can. I like to do my meditation every night before I go to bed. Some people prefer the morning, but it's my bedtime ritual. I make sure I have my journal handy, and if I'm feeling riled up, I'll journal for a while. I'll pull some divination cards and record them as I think about what they mean to me. Then, I do about twenty minutes of breath-based sitting meditation until I feel my mind go flat and calm.

The gifts that come from a spiritual practice are plentiful. It will:

- Help with mood and stress levels, significantly lowering cortisol and the stress hormone

- Balance brain chemistry

- Open your pineal gland, the location in the brain that creates psychic ability and is our connection to the Divine

- Open the energy centers, which are responsible for psychic ability and spiritual connection

- Quiet the mind so that we can be receptive to what our guides say

- Strengthen the immune system

- Create relaxation

Find something that works for you. Your guides will be so happy that you're creating an opening for them and listening. It takes discipline to stick with a spiritual practice, but the rewards will be well worth it. Spiritual practice has so many benefits for your health, your state of mind, your stress levels, and your psychic ability. If you consistently do these things—journaling, divination, meditation, or other spiritual practices—your psychic ability will grow.

The Takeaway

In this chapter, we discovered the true nature of psychic guidance and let go of some common misconceptions about the nature of psychic insights. I am sure you now realize how psychic you really are! The best way to increase your psychic acumen is to figure out which one of your psychic senses is the strongest and really pay attention to those messages. Don't forget, the psychic senses are:

- The visual sense—seeing things, usually with the inner eye

- The auditory sense—hearing our guidance as an inner conversation

- The somatic sense—feeling information in our own body

- The intuitive sense—you just *know*

- The empathic sense—getting information through feelings

- Mediumship—speaking to the dead

Once you know what your strongest psychic sense is, really pay attention to it. With time and practice, the other psychic senses will open for you as well. Learning how to trust your hits takes practice, but paying attention and beginning to act on your hits will help develop your gifts.

Remember, the best practices for further awakening your psychic gifts are keeping a psychic journal to record and interpret your hits and developing a spiritual practice for regular listening time. If you do these things with regularity, I know you will see a significant increase in your psychic ability, and this will be a huge help for your Reiki practice, as well as a wonderful advantage in your life.

In the next chapter, we are going to dive deeply into the human energy field. It will be a fun and exciting exploration of what exactly is your energy field and why you need to know about it as a Reiki practitioner.

CHAPTER 3

Your Energy Body

In this chapter, you are going to learn about the human energy field. The more Reiki you do on other people, the more you will begin to perceive their energy fields. Much as physicians must study the physical anatomy, energy medicine practitioners must study the human energy anatomy. I will also cover some practical and effective ways for Reiki practitioners to manage their energy. Learning to ground, clear, and protect yourself is essential so that you can do Reiki without carrying around unwanted energy that you picked up from your Reiki recipients. Very sensitive people will find these energy-management practices to be vital in all areas of life.

The human energy field is a complex system with three distinct parts:

- Aura, which extends beyond the physical body

- Chakras, seven energy centers located in the body

- Hara line, connects us to our life purpose

Together, they make up the energy field. The more Reiki you do, the more sensitive you will become to feeling, seeing, and perceiving these aspects. Sometimes this system is called the *subtle energy system*, *light body*, or *energy body*.

Chances are very good that you have already perceived the energy field of someone you are working on. If you have identified cold spots, energy releases, and places where energy is blocked or flowing easily, you are feeling the energy field of the person you are working on. Having a coherent and complete knowledge of the energy field will help you know what you are encountering, what it means, and what to do about it in a Reiki treatment session. You wouldn't want your surgeon to operate on you without knowing anatomy, right?

Aura Basics

At Reiki Level 1, you learn about the *aura*, which is the layers of non-physical energy that extend through and around our body. The aura changes all the time depending on our emotions, mental activity, and even our physical health. It's like a barometer, reflecting what is going on inside of you. It provides a snapshot of how you're feeling in any given moment.

The aura is made up of our life-force energy, or what some spiritual traditions call chi (or ki) or prana. This is the part of ourselves that is pure energy. The aura follows the basic contours of our physical bodies and forms a sort of energetic boundary between us and the rest of the world. Our aura tells us when someone is in our space, even if the person is not touching us. It grows larger when we're stimulated by strong emotions or are around a lot of people. The more sensitive and empathic you are, the more impacted your aura is by your environment and your interactions with others.

Your aura interacts with the auras of other people, and with the energy fields of plants, animals, and minerals, too. Someone can "rub" their feelings off onto us—we feel this all time. Some people are very sensitive to this energy, while others feel it on a more subconscious level, but everyone is affected by it.

Each of us vibrates at an energy frequency that is uniquely our own; this is our *energy signature*, or our unique vibration. It is the layer of our aura that lies close to our physical bodies. We read other people's energy signatures all the time, and usually unconsciously. Our energy attracts and repels other energies based on the principles of resonance (see "The Laws of Resonance"). *Resonance* is a concept in physics that says that everything is vibrating, down to our molecules. When something vibrates in harmony, or the same as something else, the vibrations get louder. This is opposed to the concept of *dissonance*, which states that vibrations that don't resonate with each other lower the frequency of both vibrations. In other words, like vibrations increase the amplitude of each other and unlike vibrations decrease the amplitude of each other.

Vibration is one of the ways that we measure energy flow. Physicists use the word "vibration" to describe the movement of particles to create sound waves. Energy medicine practitioners use the word "vibration" to describe chi energy movement through our body. In fact, Reiki is a form of *vibrational healing*. There are many vibrational healing methods, including homeopathy, gemstone healing, aromatherapy, sound healing, polarity therapy, and integrated energy therapy (IET).

Let's use gemstones as an example. Each type of gemstone has a unique frequency, or vibration. When we put that gemstone on a chakra, that chakra will begin to resonate with the gemstone and change its frequency to match or harmonize with the gemstone. In energy medicine, we call this process *entrainment*. That is when something with a weaker vibration (the chakra) begins to resonate with something that has a stronger vibration (the gemstone). This is fundamentally how Reiki works, too. The Reiki recipient will come into resonance with the flow of Reiki energy and the Reiki practitioner.

We certainly experience the world of vibration all the time whether we know it or not. When we say, "I don't like that person's vibe," we are reading the person's energy field and deciding if it resonates with ours. Being around someone who resonates with you makes you feel good because it raises your vibration, just as being around someone who you are out of resonance with makes you feel drained because the person lowers your vibration. It takes a lot of conscious control of our energy field to stay at our own vibration and not be affected by someone else's. The stronger someone's aura is, the more likely it is to affect yours, either negatively or positively.

We can experience this energy as color and other sensations like texture, taste, or smell. Our brain processes energy frequency through our five senses, and we perceive energetic signatures through those of our senses that are most open to us. You can go back to your psychic senses to see how you might be perceiving this energy in others. Color, texture, and odor are strongest for me. For example, I might experience someone's aura as golden in color, smooth like silk, and smelling of honey. My own energy signature is purple, smells like grapes and lavender, and feels like velvet. After doing Reiki for so many years, it is natural for me to sense people's energy this way. You will have your own way of perceiving other people's energy, depending on which of your senses are the most active. The strength of your perception will also grow with practice.

The Structure of the Aura

The aura is made up of layers, each vibrating at a different rate. The slower, denser vibrations are closest to the body, while the outer layers vibrate faster the farther they are from the body. I use a five-layer model when I'm teaching Reiki, although there are other models that have different numbers. This structure resonates most strongly with me—it's how I tend to see people's auras.

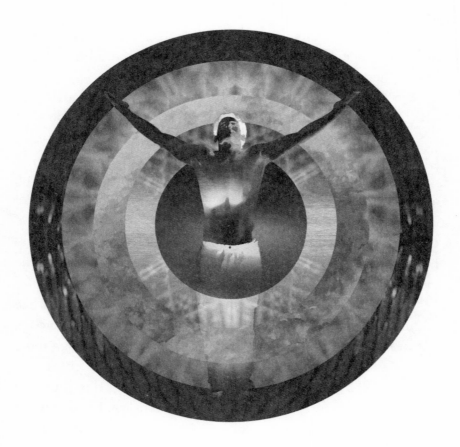

Here are the five layers I discuss when teaching others about the aura:

1. The physical layer

2. The emotional layer

3. The mental layer

4. The spiritual layer

5. The boundary layer

THE PHYSICAL LAYER

This layer is closest to the body and is the easiest one to feel when we are doing Reiki. It's only a few inches wide and starts at the edge of the physical body. It's dense and can be felt as heat just off the body. It has one color that doesn't change, and that color is different depending upon the person. This is the energy signature, which is unique to each person. We can sense physical illness or injuries in this layer of the aura. This section of the aura will feel damaged where there is physical damage in the body.

THE EMOTIONAL LAYER

The next layer beyond the physical layer is the emotional layer. It's much wider, usually about eight to twelve inches. This layer changes colors constantly according to your emotional state—kind of like a mood ring! Colors move through it quickly as we feel different emotions. It can become weakened through unresolved emotional trauma. The emotional layer of the aura is easy to damage and often appears mucky and sticky when it is filled with unprocessed emotions. People associate certain emotions with certain colors, and this partly reflects what is going on in the emotional layer of the aura.

- Red is associated with anger or lust.

- Orange is associated with sexuality, playfulness, and pleasure.

THE LAW OF RESONANCE

Resonance can be described as complementary energies that tend to vibrate like each other. Perhaps you have seen someone hit a tuning fork, and then hold an identical fork in the other hand; it begins to vibrate, too, even though the forks are not touching and the second one hadn't been struck. Like tunes itself to like, naturally and automatically.

Have you ever met someone and right away you just couldn't stand them? That person's energy did not resonate with yours—it was dissonant and repelled you instead of attracting you. We feel it energetically when we have a lack of harmony with someone. We feel these energies unconsciously and automatically, whether we know anything about our subtle energy system or not.

Reiki is a form of vibrational medicine, which works according to the law of resonance, like this:

- When we need healing, our energy vibrates at a lower frequency and is much weaker than it should be.

- Reiki is aligned with the Universal Life Force energy and is vibrating very strongly with the energy of unconditional love.

- When something vibrates strongly, it pulls other frequencies in to match it. This is called entrainment.

- Being drawn into harmony with the vibration of Universal Life Force energy and love brings healing to us.

When we give or receive Reiki, we begin to entrain or resonate with Reiki energy. Gemstones, crystals, homeopathic remedies, and essential oils also have strong healing frequencies, and it is because of the process of entrainment that these items are often used by Reiki practitioners and other vibrational or energy healers.

- Yellow is associated with thinking and mental activity.

- Green is associated with healing.

- Pink is love.

- Blue can be associated with sadness and grief or with peacefulness and serenity.

- Purple is associated with faith and connection to spirit.

- Pea green is associated with jealousy.

- Brown is associated with resentment and disempowerment.

- Black is associated with ill health and depression.

The emotional layer of the aura holds all our emotional wounds, which can look like bruising and feel like slimy muck.

THE MENTAL LAYER

This is the layer of our aura associated with our thoughts, and it lies outside the emotional layer. The mental layer of the aura usually looks yellow or gold and is much thinner than the emotional layer. It's usually just a few inches wide, although if someone is thinking a lot, it expands. Accessing this layer allows us to clean up our thinking and correct our mistaken thoughts and beliefs. Sometimes illnesses spring from our faulty and wounded thinking and we can perceive the imprint of that here. For example, the thought *I am not worthy* will leave behind an imprint in the mental layer of your aura. That thought might then create a feeling of shame, self-disgust, anger, or fear in the emotional layer. It will look like a bruise there. This, in turn, can trickle through our system and create a problem in the corresponding part of the body. In this case, probably around the solar plexus chakra. (You'll learn more about chakras later in this chapter.)

THE SPIRITUAL LAYER

Sometimes called the *light body*, the spiritual layer of the aura is our interface with the spiritual world. It is right within the outer boundary of the aura. Your guides connect to you here, and here is where your own soul connects to the Divine. This layer is radiant and luminous. Although it often appears as pure white light, it can be any color. In people who have spent a long time developing their connection to spirit, this layer is very wide and vibrant.

The spiritual layer holds all our past-life wounding, which some call our *karma*. It's a tough layer to heal! The best healing for this layer is a strong spiritual practice. In general, Reiki and other vibrational medicines work best on our aura's physical, emotional, mental, and boundary layers. The spiritual layer of the aura is very hard to work on. There are some healers who can impact the light body during a healing. Just being in the persence of a real spiritual master can change your light body. Sometimes a guru will give you *shakipat*, which is when they put their hands on you to consciously and radically shift your light body as a blessing to you. This will have an extreme effect on you, perhaps even putting you in a higher state of consciousness.

The "hugging saint," known as Amma, is an example of such a guru. She can change your light body with just a hug, which is her way of giving a blessing. Spiritual practice is the best way to change the light body, which is another fantastic reason to be committed to a spiritual practice.

THE BOUNDARY LAYER

This layer is like a membrane that covers the entire energy field, demarcating your energy field from the rest of the world. This is the layer that acts as a protector, keeping the energy of your aura with you. It's looks like a very fine mesh or screen, golden in color. For people who are nonempathic, the mesh is very tightly woven and almost solid. The boundary layer of empaths, on the other hand, has a porous quality, which explains a lot about why they feel so sensitive. The boundary layer is like your skin. It's liable to get damaged, ripped, or worn thin, and it frequently needs repair. An unrepaired hole in this layer of your aura can seriously affect your whole being, as all kinds of energy, both good *and* bad, can get into your system through this opening.

Physical and emotional trauma can shred this layer of your aura, making it weak, so it's important to do whatever healing work you need to do to heal up any unresolved trauma. Empaths leak energy through this layer, as well as absorb other people's energy. If you're highly empathic, learning to strengthen this layer of your aura is essential. More on exactly how to do that later in this chapter.

HEALING YOUR TRAUMA

If you have had major trauma in your life, you need to handle that. I have noticed that many people who are drawn to the healing arts often have experienced severe trauma, and many identify with the "wounded healer" archetype. People with trauma in their past make excellent healers, but it's essential that they heal their own trauma along the way. Nearly everyone has some trauma in their past, but for some of us the traumas are profound, such as the death of a family member; divorce; illness; incest; or physical, sexual, and emotional abuse.

If you know you have serious trauma in yourself that needs healing, I recommend a holistic approach that works on the levels of your being, including the body, emotions, and your energetic and spiritual selves. We need to receive healing work on all these levels to heal deep trauma. This can include:

- Body work, such as cranial sacral work, chiropractic, and myofascial release therapy

- Emotional work, such as all the different variations of psychotherapy, breath work, or emotional freedom technique

- Energy work, such as Reiki, acupuncture, and polarity therapy

- Spiritual work, such as past-life and shamanic work, and, of course, regular spiritual practice

When we engage in our own healing work at all these levels, we can heal even terrible trauma. It's essential to do this work.

Perceiving the Aura

The aura is not all that hard to perceive. Many times, we perceive people's auras without knowing that we are doing it. Have you ever been listening to someone speak in a class, or maybe in church, and noticed a white or lightly colored outline around the person's head or body? *That's* the aura. I can teach most people how to sense an aura in about ten minutes. The following two exercises will teach you two different ways to do this.

LEARNING TO PERCEIVE AURAS

If you want to learn to perceive an aura, you need someone to practice with. Ask that person to stand in front of a white wall. Stand a few yards away from the person. Begin by looking directly at the person and squinting. Soft focusing our eyes can help us see energy. Then use your peripheral vision: turn your head and look at the person out of the corner of your eye. People with a strong visual psychic ability will see colors or an outline of white light around the person they're looking at.

Next, try closing your eyes and continue "looking" at the person. Most people "see" better psychically when their eyes are closed. Try asking yourself if you know what color the person's energy field is. You might hear the answer as a voice in your head, or you may just know, feel, or sense it.

Keep practicing this and you'll learn to perceive auras in no time! Some people have an easy, natural ability to do this, and other people need to practice a little more. Also, the more you do Reiki on other people, the more this ability will naturally increase. Many people who practice Reiki frequently will just spontaneously start seeing colors around their clients.

HOT HANDS EXERCISE

For those of you who are more feelers and somatic psychics, try this exercise that helps you practice feeling energy with your hands.

Rub your hands together until you feel some heat. Hold your palms together and slowly pull them apart until you feel a sensation like heat.

Then, starting with your hands far away from each other, slowly bring them together until you feel something. It helps to move your hands around in circles, like you are making a ball of energy. You may feel heat, tingling, or resistance. The resistance feels a bit like putting together the two wrong ends of a pair of magnets.

You might feel it when your hands are a foot apart, or you might not feel it until your hands are very close together. Try it with someone else, too. If you stand facing each other, you can start with your hands up and touching each other. Then slowly move your hands apart until you feel sensation. Try moving your hands around in circles near your partner's hands and noticing how the sensation changes.

Once you've played with that awhile, you can try feeling your aura above your chest or your belly. Start with your hands out and bring them toward your body until you feel a sensation in your hands.

Now that you understand more about your aura, we are going to learn some easy and practical ways to manage your energy field. These tips and techniques will assist you in keeping your energy field clear and repairing any damage to the outer boundary layer of your aura.

Managing Your Aura

As Reiki practitioners, it's essential that we understand, heal, and manage our own energy systems. This starts with managing our own aura. We experience huge benefits when we can manage our energy and huge problems can arise when we don't.

The aura acts as our first line of defense against unwanted psychic, emotional, and physical energy coming into our systems. It's literally the boundary between us and the rest of the world—the energetic equivalent of skin. People who have a weak outer edge to their energy field get sick a lot. Just like a cut in your skin can lead to an infection, holes and tears in the outer edge of your energy field can lead to a weakened immune system.

The aura gets damaged easily and needs to be healed regularly for us to maintain a healthy boundary with the world. When it's injured, we leak energy, leaving us feeling defenseless and drained.

Unresolved trauma is the main culprit when it comes to a chronically damaged aura, but unhealthy living habits contribute as well.

Most of us have poor energy habits, just as we often have poor eating habits, but taking regular care of the energy system is a good *energy habit* to develop. When you're first learning to manage your aura, daily meditation and visualization are key. Since our auras respond easily to our thoughts and intentions, visualizing and meditating are very effective ways to change your aura.

DAILY AURA-CLEARING MEDITATION

Sit comfortably with your feet on the ground and your arms and legs uncrossed. You can sit cross-legged if you like, but it's easier to ground when the bottoms of our feet are on the ground. Get your spine as upright as you can.

Begin with a deep breath. Imagine that you are breathing light in the top of your head. Fill your heart and your belly with that light. On the exhale breath, release energy down your spine, down your legs, and into the ground through the bottoms of your feet. You can imagine that you are releasing all that you are holding on to on that exhale. Release all your own emotions and all the emotions and energy that you have picked up from other people, too. Release everything down into the ground with the exhale. (Don't worry, the earth knows how to compost this energy.) Do this sequence a few times until you feel like you are clear and grounded.

Now, concentrate on the outer edge of your energy field. Since our auras respond very well to our imagination and visualization, you can imagine, pretend, or visual this. Once you have visualized the outer edge of your energy field, you can make it more solid, like an eggshell or a crystal ball. Shine it up.

Then, program the outer edge of your energy field to only let in positive and supportive energy. It should be semipermeable, like the membrane of a cell. Nonsupportive energy stays on the other side and nothing crosses this boundary without your permission.

Take another final inhale breath to add as much light to your aura as you can and exhale again, releasing any extra energy down your legs and into the ground.

Do this entire exercise as many times as you need to throughout the day.

Our daily habits either support or hurt our auras, and it will probably not surprise you that the same habits that support our physical and mental health also support our energetic health. The following are some of the things that can weaken our auras:

- Unresolved physical or emotional trauma

- Poor diet

- No exercise

- Drugs and alcohol

- Poor sleep

- Stress and worry

- EMF radiation (electromagnetic fields from TVs, microwaves, computers, cell phones, X-rays)

- Unhealthy relationships or too much isolation

- Hating your job or any important aspect of your life

- Clutter and mess in your environment

- Anger and resentment

- Victim attitude and blaming others

The following are some of the things that can strengthen our auras:

- Healthy diet

- Physical exercise

- Sufficient resting and sleeping

- Positive thinking

- Breathing deeply from the belly

- Spending time outside

- A spiritual practice that includes prayer and meditation

- Physical spiritual practices like yoga, tai chi, and qigong

- A clean, clutter-free environment

- Handling your emotions as they come up

- Healing body work (like Reiki and massage)

- Doing emotional healing work like therapy

- Choosing a life that you love

It's easy to see what makes the aura healthy and what damages it. Genuine ways of taking care of ourselves also support the aura. Shadow comforts and addictions weaken the aura. If you feel truly good about what you're doing, it's probably good for the aura. If you feel guilty, yucky, or conflicted about something you're doing, it's probably damaging your aura.

When the aura is weak, especially the boundary layer, it can have a profoundly negative impact on your physical, mental, emotional, and spiritual health. When your aura is damaged, you'll be:

- Depleted and exhausted

- Depressed and anxious

- Prone to illness

Drugs, alcohol, and a poor diet are among the worst offenders, as is trauma of any kind. It's very important to clear up any lingering trauma by going to therapy and working with healers. Reiki is a big help here. On top of that, you can do specific practices, including the guided meditations and energy-management exercises that we will learn later in this book. Check out the link http://www.newharbin ger.com/41214 on the New Harbinger website for access to a guided audio meditation that is designed specifically to keep your entire energy field healthy and strong.

All the electrical energy that we have in our world is tough on our energy field. Fluorescent lights, TV, video games, computers, microwaves, cell phones, and other Wi-Fi-enabled devices are all big culprits. That's why you start feeling yucky if you spend all day in front of the TV or a computer. Going shopping or to the mall is tough on the aura as well, since it's the perfect storm of being in crowds, sensory stimuli, and electromagnetic energy, all of which tax the aura. If you are especially empathic or psychically sensitive, crowds, stimuli, and electromagnetic energy will fray your aura particularly fast. Nature, gentle movement, and fresh air are good energy antidotes.

Now that you have learned the ins and outs of what your aura is and how to take care of it, it's time to learn about the next part of our energy field, the chakras.

Chakra Basics

Chakras are the energy centers located in the body, and chances are you have already felt or perceived these energy centers either in yourself or others as you have been doing Reiki. Your chakras each represent an aspect of your life. They are a fabulous lens through which to look at your actual life and see what is happening in a concrete way. Chakras are where people's problems show up, since they hold both the potential and the wounds for those areas of life. We are also going to discover how to treat blocks in the chakras and how this corresponds to health issues in the body.

Chakra is a Sanskrit word that means "wheel," but chakras are so much more than spinning wheels of light. When we do Reiki, we start at the head and work down the body, focusing on the chakras and releasing blocked energy or replacing lost energy in each chakra as needed. Our goal is to balance the chakras individually, but also to balance them as a system.

Each chakra is associated with a color, a location in the body, and the area of your life that it governs. The chakras are also three-dimensional, like funnels, and chakras two through six have both a front and back aspect to them. They plug into the *hara line*, the midline current of energy that runs up and down our spine. Chakras one (the root) and seven (the crown) are connected to each other through the hara line.

Chakras become blocked when we have an unresolved trauma or unprocessed emotions lodged in them. If something bad happens to us, our chakras can get stuck holding on to that experience until we release it. Chakras get blocked in two different ways. They can be *excessive*, which means that they have too much energy running through them. Or, they can be *deficient*, which means they are undercharged and don't have enough energy running through them. Both are considered blockages.

When the chakras are functioning well, they allow us to be fluid and to live in the moment, without running old programs from the past. This creates both relaxation and power in us. We are in the moment, feeling open and curious without anxiety, and we are also able to act decisively with power when we need to.

It pays to clear up your chakras! When we clear our chakras, we release from them old wounds and stuck energy and emotions, which allows us to be fully present in the moment. This concept of the chakras will be useful as you begin to do Reiki. You may start experiencing the chakras of the people you are working on, so you need a context right away.

Chakra One

Located at the base of your spine, chakra one is also called the *root chakra*. It's red and it is the chakra of your physical body. It governs your physical health and your basic survival needs. People with a strong first chakra are very good at managing the physical world. They tend to have a nice house, good health, and money in the bank. They handle their survival needs with ease. People with a deficient first chakra, on the other hand, may have poor health and struggle with basic survival needs. An excessive first chakra creates clutter in your environment, excess weight on the body, and an inability to handle change in your life.

When this chakra is open and functioning well, you will be grounded, feel secure, and have courage. Because it's the survival chakra it is blocked by fear. People who grew up in unsafe households or in poverty will carry a wound in this chakra. Clearing and healing this chakra allows you to better manage your life in the world. Here are some actions you can take to clear and heal chakra one:

- Take care of your body by eating right, exercising, and getting plenty of sleep.

- Manage the details of your life, such as paying your bills, maintaining your possessions, and generally taking care of day-to-day business.

- Clear clutter from your environment

To treat chakra one in Reiki, we work on the hips, knees, legs and feet.

Chakra Two

Chakra two is located just below your navel and is associated with the color orange. It governs our basic emotions, such as anger, sadness, and happiness. It's where we feel our passion for life and for sex. It's often blocked, since most people have plenty of repressed emotional and sexual energy. When the chakra is open, we flow with life, feel pleasure, and let our emotions guide us in a healthy way.

When this chakra is deficient, we are closed off to all emotions, pleasure, and sexuality, and we are generally repressed. An excessive second chakra means we are swamped by our feelings and chase pleasure in unhealthy ways.

This chakra is opened when you partake in healthy pleasure and is blocked by guilt. Clearing and managing this chakra allows you to be guided by your emotions and enjoy healthy pleasure and passions in your life. Here are some actions you can take to clear and heal the second chakra:

- Find a safe and comfortable way to express your emotions, such as journaling or working with a therapist to let your emotions flow.

- Do fluid movement like yoga, dance, walking, or swimming.

- Prioritize things that you feel passionate about and that you love doing.

- Look for the pleasure in everyday moments.

In Reiki, we treat chakra two by working on the lower back at the sacrum and the lower belly.

Chakra Three

Chakra three is located in the solar plexus, and it is associated with a bright, sunny yellow color. It rules our sense of personal power and self-esteem. When it's open, we feel capable, determined, and disciplined, and we like ourselves. Our feeling of self-worth allows us to say no and set appropriate boundaries.

When this chakra is deficient, we have low self-esteem and have trouble accomplishing things. We let people walk all over us and can't say no or set boundaries. An excessive third chakra means we might walk all over others and be bossy, arrogant, and self-centered.

This chakra is opened when you work toward and accomplish your goals and is blocked by shame. Clearing and managing this chakra allows you to live confidently with good self-esteem and easily accomplish goals. To clear and heal this chakra:

- Do self-esteem work in therapy.

- Set boundaries by saying no when you need to.

- Strengthen your core through yoga or Pilates.

- Set goals and accomplish them.

To treat the third chakra in Reiki, we focus on the solar plexus and midback.

Chakra Four

Chakra four is located in the heart area and is associated with the color green. It rules our relationships and self-love. It also holds higher-frequency emotions, like joy and compassion. When it's open, we love ourselves and have healthy, satisfying relationships with others.

A deficient fourth chakra means that our hearts are shut down to loving ourselves and others. With an excessive fourth chakra, we get mired in codependent, dysfunctional relationships.

The heart chakra is opened by cultivating love, forgiveness, and compassion and is blocked by unexpressed grief. Clearing and managing this chakra allows you to love yourself fully and live with a heart full of compassion for others. We forgive and release the past and allow ourselves to love again without fear. Here are some actions you can take to clear and heal the fourth chakra:

- Practice loving yourself; try self-loving affirmations. (For example, "I love and accept myself exactly as I am.")

- Do forgiveness work and let go of past hurts.

- Clean up any dysfunctional relationships with couples therapy.

- Practice feeling compassion for all of humanity. (Doing Reiki is a great way to do this.)

To treat the fourth chakra in Reiki, we focus on the center of the chest and the back between the shoulder blades.

Chakra Five

Chakra five is the throat chakra. It is located in the throat and its color is sky blue. The throat chakra handles our ability to communicate through speaking, writing, or other creative pursuits. It's also our ability to listen, since communication is a two-way street. When this chakra is open, we can speak the truth of our hearts and minds with ease and listen to others.

When it's deficient, we stammer and stutter and are unable to express what's in our hearts. An excessive fifth chakra will have you interrupting and speaking a lot but saying very little and unable to listen. You can hear the quality of someone's fifth chakra by listening to the tone and quality of the person's voice. Deficient folks have mousy voices that you can barely hear, and excessive people have booming voices that drown out others.

Speaking our truth clearly and creatively opens the throat chakra, and it is blocked when we lie or stay silent. Clearing and managing this chakra allows you to fully say what you need to say and to express yourself through creative endeavors. Here are some actions you can take to clear and heal chakra five:

- Speak your heart's truth in kind and thoughtful ways.

- Practice the Buddhist precept of Right Speech, which includes asking yourself before you speak: *Is it true? Is it kind? Is it necessary?*

- Actively listen to other people without interrupting and arguing.

- Chant, sing, and speak mantras.

- Engage in creative expression, such as journaling, creative writing, music, and art.

In Reiki, to treat the fifth chakra, we hover at the front of the neck (since most people dislike being touched there) and touch the back of the neck.

Chakra Six

Chakra six is the brow chakra, and it is located at the center of the forehead. Its color is deep indigo blue. It's a tricky chakra to work with, since it governs our mind and how we think, as well as how we see ourselves in the world. It's our viewpoint. When it's open, we are open-minded and see things from everyone's perspective.

When it's deficient, our minds are shut down to new ideas or to seeing other people's points of view; we are literally closed-minded.

With an excessive sixth chakra we overthink everything, losing ourselves in overanalysis and overidentifying with our thoughts in the classic motto of overthinkers: "I think, therefore I am."

The brow chakra is opened when we learn new things and expand our point of view; it is blocked by tightly held illusions and rigid mind-sets. Clearing and managing this chakra allows you to see your place in the world and to take in new ideas. When this chakra is functioning properly, your mind is flexible and adaptable and easily sees things from many viewpoints. Here are some actions you can take to clear and heal chakra six:

- Learn to examine your thoughts to see if they are true or not.

- Expose yourself to new people, ideas, and situations.

- Open your worldview by trying new things, like traveling.

- Clean up negative and rigid thinking patterns through methods like neurolinguistic programming, which is a powerful psychological tool that uses conscious changes in our language to change the way that we think about things.

In Reiki, to treat the sixth chakra, we focus on the forehead and on the occiput (back of the skull).

Chakra Seven

Chakra seven is called the *crown chakra* because it's located at the top of the head. It is associated with either violet or white, and it manages our connection to Divine energy, including our guides. When it is open, we experience infinite possibility and we have the experience of "I can do anything!" We are connected to universal consciousness.

When it's deficient, we feel disconnected from the Divine, lack faith, and suffer from spiritual depression. An excessive seventh chakra puts everything in the hands of the Divine and disconnects us from our personal responsibilities in a "my angels will do it for me" kind of way.

This chakra is opened by faith and blocked by attachment to the material world. Clearing and managing this chakra allows you to feel guided by a higher power and to connect with that guidance on a regular basis. Here are some actions you can take to clear and heal chakra seven:

- Practice meditation. (This is by far the best way to keep the seventh chakra open.)

- Maintain any form of spiritual practice, including prayer, yoga, or chanting.

- Worship in a spiritual community, like a church, temple, or mosque.

- Continue to open yourself to possibilities and keep a positive mind-set.

To treat this chakra with Reiki, we send Reiki to the top of the head, hovering the hands over the top of the head.

Each chakra represents a very real and tangible aspect of our being. Sometimes my clients come to a Reiki session and ask me to fix and clear all their chakras, as if that would magically erase all the problems in their lives. I wish it were so easy! Since what is happening in the chakra is a reflection of what is happening in your life, a Reiki healer can clear and balance your chakras, which will then give you some openness and leverage in that aspect of your life. However, it takes deeper healing work to truly bring about lasting change in our lives and our chakras. It can be the work of a lifetime, but it's good work!

When we have experienced trauma and something wounds us in a particular area of our life, it creates a block or wound in the corresponding chakra. Doing a Reiki treatment on the blocked chakra will help loosen up stuck energy in that chakra, as well as that aspect of the person's life. That's where the lasting change comes in.

The Takeaway

In this chapter, you learned some crucial material about the nature of your energy field, including the aura and the chakras. As Reiki practitioners, it's very important to understand the anatomy of your energy field and how to manage your aura so that you can live, work, and do your Reiki sessions without compromising your energy field.

In summary, it's good to remember that:

- Your aura has five layers. If you practice, you will easily learn how to perceive these layers when you are doing Reiki.

- It's vital to take care of your aura by doing daily aura-clearing meditations.

- Your chakras present actual parts of your life, and you hold unhealed trauma in them.

- As you clear out your chakras, your life will get better!

In the next chapter, I'll talk about managing your energy in ways that make it safe for you to do Reiki. There'll be a bit more energy anatomy—I'll talk about the hara line—but the focus will be on attending to yourself in a way that will allow you to channel healing energy without compromising your own energetic field. This is important for anyone who is embarking on a Reiki practice, but it's essential for those who are highly empathic or psychically sensitive. You need extra care and attention so that you can learn to manage your energy while you are doing Reiki. I think you will find that the skills and practices you learn will also help you in the rest of your life.

CHAPTER 4

Energy Management

This chapter is about energy management for all Reiki practitioners, since attending to our own energetic needs makes us all better healers. We'll be specifically discussing the needs of empaths, who are most in need of good energy-management tools.

As I mentioned in chapter 1, being empathic is much more than just being emotionally sensitive. Empathy is a bit like sympathy in that it's the ability to put yourself in someone else's shoes. When we are sympathetic, we feel *for* people. When we are empathic, we feel *with* them; our bodies, hearts, minds, and souls experience some part of what the other is going through. Research shows that the more empathic people are, the more kindness, compassion, and generosity they exhibit. People with deeply empathic natures are almost unable to commit acts of violence.

Nearly all humans are empathic to a degree—it's just part of who we are as beings. We feel each other's feelings and share each other's energy. As with any trait, some of us are more gifted with empathy than others. As with any gift, it can be both a blessing and a burden. When we don't take precautions, even the blessed part starts to feel like a burden. This happened to my student Ashley.

❀ *Ashley's Story* ❀
On the Edge of Burnout

Ashley is a very gifted energy healer. She is a social worker and Reiki practitioner and felt called to take her work to hospices to assist people who are dying, as well as their families. Then she got sick. Her thyroid was off and she was exhausted and suffering from digestive problems and adrenal fatigue. She was also feeling deeply burned-out. She was desperate and in bad shape.

"Lisa, I love the work I do, I truly love it," she said. "I know I'm good at it, but it's killing me. I come home from a case and I'm wiped out. I get migraines all the time and my joints are swollen. The doctors tell me its fibromyalgia. The exhaustion I feel is so bad that sometimes I can't get off the couch for days." Ashley continued, "I can't afford to be down like this! I have a life. I have kids and a husband who need me, and I feel terrible that I can't show up for them right now. My work is just sucking me dry."

"I know how tough it is when you're so sensitive and you spend your days healing others," I responded. "It's a lot to handle."

"Tell me about it," Ashley said. "Being in hospitals and nursing homes is very hard for me. I can't process all the feelings that are coming at me. I just suck up all the pain and misery that everyone else is feeling, and when you're working with people who are dying, there's plenty of that. I feel everyone's feelings for them, and they are painful feelings, all day long, every day. The worst thing is that I don't know anyone to talk to about this. It's not like you can just explain this to people. I feel like such a freak, like there is really something wrong with me. Yesterday, I actually wondered if I was going crazy!"

"You're not crazy," I reassured her. "You would be surprised how many people are empaths like you. It's a big club."

Ashley responded, "I know you say it's a gift, but honestly it feels like a huge curse. I think I'm going to have to quit my job! I can't keep doing this."

I wrote this book because lots of my Reiki students, like Ashley, are strong empaths and psychically gifted people. It's why they're drawn to Reiki in the first place, and why they are so good at it once they've begun learning and practicing. Learning and practicing Reiki will inevitably make you even *more* empathic. This is a good thing, and it can also be overwhelming. It became clear to me that some training aimed at helping people manage their empathic energy would make them better Reiki practitioners. And, it would also help them live more happy and sustainable lives.

If you are an empath and haven't had training on how to manage your energy, it's very likely that you suffer from *empathic overload*. This is a combination of fatigue, anxiety, and health issues that come from being chronically drained of life-force energy. Empaths have a difficult time holding on to their own energy because their energy fields are so leaky. They overgive and have trouble saying no to other people. They often have weakened immune systems due to the porous nature of the energy fields.

The outer edge of our energy field is connected to our immune system, and when that is weak and shaky, we are not only subject to people's energy penetrating our energy field, but we can also pick up every passing bug that is going around. Empaths are also very sensitive to electromagnetic radiation, which studies have recently confirmed has a negative impact on our autoimmune system. Empaths are also prone to anxiety when they think about leaving their homes, especially if they are already tired.

Ashley's story is very typical for empaths and shows the classic symptoms of empathic overload. All empaths are drawn to helping, healing, and service work, and that often puts us right in the line of fire. Learning energy management and deep psychological and spiritual healing give you back the power that comes with your gift.

There are seven pieces to becoming an empowered empath. The first is just pure acceptance of your gift. The second is understanding just how energy transfer happens for empaths—it's powerful and can be destructive to you if not managed with care. The next four are energy-management practices: grounding, clearing, replenishment, and boundary maintenance. The seventh is making an ongoing commitment to healing from psychological, spiritual, and energetic wounds. We'll discuss the first five in this chapter and the other two a bit later. Let's start with acceptance.

Accepting Your Gift

Being an empath is like having the range of an opera singer, except the range refers to emotional notes not musical ones. We can hit all the high notes and all the low notes, too. We must truly accept, embrace, and develop our emotional gift if we don't want to squander it.

You Were Born This Way

Empaths are born and not made. Being an empath is a core soul quality: if we're empathic now, we have been for most of our lifetime. Of course, we can and do become more empathic over time, but I have never met an empath who just suddenly woke up one day with this gift. Some empaths use their gift to navigate rocky childhoods. It can be an adaptive strategy if you're born into a family with unpredictable caregivers. Some lucky empathic kids are valued and supported for their gifts, but often, empaths have learned to be ashamed of our sensitivity within our family systems.

CONNECTING WITH YOUR INNER CHILD

Take a moment right now to think back on your childhood. Ask yourself how your family responded to your sensitivity.

- Was it praised and accepted?

- Was it ignored?

- Was it treated with fear and distrust?

Consider what words were used with you. Did you get the message to "get a thicker skin" or were you told you were too sensitive? Perhaps you were told, "Quit crying or I will give you something to cry about." Families often react more negatively toward empathic boys than empathic girls. There are still strong cultural norms against little boys who are "too" sensitive and emotional.

Consider what happened to you in school. How was it with your teachers, and what happened on the playground? As we look at this childhood programming, we can begin to see why we reject this gift in ourselves.

Take a moment to comfort the child in you and give yourself permission to be as sensitive and empathic as you can be, knowing this is one of your most powerful gifts for the world. Feel free to give yourself a lot of Reiki as you are doing this. Try one hand on your heart and the other hand on your belly and let the Reiki energy flow into you. Breath in unconditional love for yourself with each breath.

Empaths are often told that we're too emotional and sensitive, and that we should toughen up. Katrina's story is typical.

❀ *Katrina's Story* ❀
The Overly Sensitive Child

I always knew I was different. I felt like I didn't belong and had to hide who I was to fit in. When I was a kid, I cried about everything. I cried at TV commercials. I cried when other people cried. I used to get teased for being that way—tormented, actually. I grew up being called oversensitive and told to get a thicker skin. It got to the point where I just avoided everyone and stayed home a lot. I pretended to be like everyone else, but I always felt like I was a crazy.

The shame we learn about our perceived weakness (which is actually our great strength), combined with the energetic drain of feeling all the feelings all the time, puts empaths at risk of anxiety and depression. Empaths can resort to alcohol and drugs to try and turn off their sensitivities and shut down their feelings. They may feel there is something wrong with them—that they are weak, over-sensitive, and, to top it all off, crazy!

You're Not Crazy

It's very important to understand that you're not crazy, broken, or defective in any way. There's nothing wrong with you except that you were not taught how to manage your emotions, energy field, and sensitivities.

Empaths can suffer from all different kinds of anxiety, including ambient (free-floating) anxiety and social anxiety. In some cases, empaths can become afraid to leave their homes and go out into the world. The depression that empaths feel is often linked to their difficulty being out in the world. It's depressing to be unable to interact in the world the way others do and not to be able to live your life's purpose. Those empaths who follow their calling into jobs such as nursing or teaching are also at risk of depression since these professions can put untrained, unshielded empaths directly into energetically challenging situations.

HEALING ANXIETY AND DEPRESSION

If you feel like you have anxiety and depression that you can't manage, it's very important to get help. Practice the energy-management exercises in this book. They will begin to heal and stabilize your delicate energy systems. Counseling is an important healing modality that helps us heal from past wounds, as does learning to accept ourselves. Good counseling will teach you how to manage the flow of your emotions rather than getting consumed by them.

Don't forget to do some self-healing Reiki! Healing modalities such as acupuncture and reflexology are very effective, too. Recent research has shown that both exercise and meditation are wonderful at relieving both anxiety and depression. It comes down to having a consistent self-care routine and doing deep inner-healing work to clear up any lingering emotional wounds. Inner peace and the tranquility of self-acceptance are the rewards of doing this difficult but necessary inner work.

It's good to accept that empathy, psychic insight, intuition, and healing all go together, and then to find a way to celebrate these wonderful gifts instead of trying to throw them back to the creator. Once you accept your psychic gifts, they may manifest in a completely unique way, giving you the perfect tools for your life's purpose. You can either explore these gifts or reject them, but I highly recommend that you learn to use them. This requires training and dedication since we must practice if we want to master any new skill. I strongly recommend getting the training, since sometime psychics who reject their gifts can suffer in needless ways.

Claim Your Power

Depression and anxiety can dissolve when empaths learn the skills that allow them to fulfill their life's purpose. Shame and feelings of weakness and unworthiness also dissolve when we embrace our gift and learn to use it safely. The foundational practices laid out in this chapter will give you a stronger energy field and better boundaries, and they are very effective at helping you better manage being in the world—and even begin to enjoy it! That's how it worked out for Ashley.

❀ *Ashley's Story* ❀
Becoming Empowered as an Empath

When Ashley called me, sounding so defeated and desperate, I knew I could help her. What a crime it would be for this amazing healer to have to give up her career because she couldn't manage her empathy. The world needs all the healers it can get!

Ashley and I worked together for a few months to get her healthy, off the couch, and back in action. I helped her in two ways. First, she simply learned how to manage her energy field. She learned:

How to ground herself and stay in her body while she was working

To tighten her boundaries so she was not accidentally leaking energy

How to clear the emotions that she picked up from other people, so that she wasn't carrying them around

How to replenish and refill herself

These steps are uncomplicated, easily learned, and very effective.

The second area we tackled together included the tougher stuff. We had to work at a deep level to help her manage her past wounds, breached boundaries, and painful relationships. Learning how to say no and not overgive was a crucial skill for

*her to learn. Ultimately, she learned to nourish and nurture
herself the same way she nourishes and nurtures her clients, so
that her inner well of energy was always full. Then giving to
others became a joy.*

*A few months after that first call, she called me again, this
time full of joy and vibrancy. She was off the couch and back
into life. She felt strong and dynamic, and that her job was giving
her energy instead of sucking it out of her. She faithfully practiced
the aura-strengthening exercises so she had more energy for her
family. Her marriage improved and her husband was very
grateful to have his wife back in action.*

The good news is that learning how to strengthen your energy
field is easy to do. We're going to use guided meditations to do it;
they're quick and easy and make a *big* difference right away. We will
be learning a lot more of these in the next chapter, but here is an
easy one to start with. It teaches both grounding and clearing.

THE REIKI WATERFALL EXERCISE

- Sit or stand with your back straight and push your feet into
  the floor.

- Concentrate on the long bones of your body. We can ground
  by feeling into our bones, since they are the most solid part
  of us. Connect to the Reiki energy by imagining a waterfall
  of light flowing down over your head. As this Universal Life
  Force energy flows over you and through you, use it to wash
  away anything you picked up from other people and anything of your own that you are ready to let go of.

- Finish by putting your hands on your heart and breathing
  into your heart. This reconnects you to your heart and is very
  helpful if you feel like you have lost yourself in overgiving to
  others.

You should feel grounded, clear, and reconnected to yourself after
this exercise. Do it as often as necessary.

THE GIFT OF EMPATHY

It's tough being an empath, but it's not all bad! I love giving empaths the good news that there's also much that's wonderful about it. Here is a list of some of the superpowers of your empathic gift:

- ❀ A kind, compassionate heart and the desire to be of service.

- ❀ A deeply emotional nature and a wide range of emotions.

- ❀ The ability to connect with others at a very deep level. This comes with a profound need for intimacy and deep connection.

- ❀ Amazing sensitivity to and insight into how others are feeling.

- ❀ A natural ability to heal. All empaths are healers! We each have a unique way of doing it.

- ❀ Powerful psychic and intuitive abilities.

When these beautiful qualities are combined in one person, it creates a soul who is uniquely qualified to make a difference in the world and to help people connect deeply. This is the gift of empathy.

Energy and the Empath

Empaths have a natural way of doing healing work for other people, and usually we do it unconsciously, in what is called an *energy transfer*. We'll talk more about this later in this section, but first let's learn about the mechanics of physical and emotional empathy.

Physical Empathy

When I do energy healing sessions for people and put my hands on them, I can feel in *my* body what they're feeling in *their* body. This is called *physical empathy*. For example, if my client has pain in the back, then I'll feel a twinge in my back in the same place.

Physical empathy is very good if you work hands-on with people. All good massage therapists and body workers have this ability, which is how they know exactly where to put their hands on you. However, if physical empathy happens outside of a healing context, without good energy management, it can be a nuisance. You might inadvertently pick up the headache of someone you are sitting next to. You can end up walking away from everyone you meet and keeping their aches and pains!

Clearing this unwanted energy from our system is one of the most important things you can learn, especially when doing Reiki. This is how you walk away from a Reiki session without taking your client's pain home with you. We need to learn how to tell if a particular sensation belongs to you or the person that you are working on.

There are two ways to do this. You can ask yourself, *Is this my sensation or theirs?* You might get an easy yes or no answer this way. You could hear the answer, see it, or just know it, depending on the nature of your psychic and intuitive gifts. Or, you can ask the person, "Hey, how is your lower back today?" If the person answers, "It's killing me, how did you know?" then you'll know the twinge you felt was your client's. It's quite beneficial to practice both ways of assessment. Asking yourself and then getting confirmation from the person will help build your confidence in your intuitive hits. You can also practice this in your daily life, independent of doing Reiki. If you feel something in the presence of another person, try it. Ask yourself, *How is my head feeling? Is it my sensation or the person next to me?* If you know the person in question or feel comfortable inquiring, you can ask directly, "How are you feeling?" Once you find out it's coming from the other person, you can practice clearing it from your own body.

I have enough practice with physical empathy and energy clearing that it takes me maybe a minute or two to identify it, check in with my client, and then clear it. To get rid of the sensation, practice *flushing* it down your grounding cord with your breath. Review the Quick Energy Clearing Technique exercise below for more detailed instruction on how to do this. Don't hold on to it!

QUICK ENERGY CLEARING TECHNIQUE

This technique is quick and very effective and will help you practice clearing your energy. It's beneficial to use after you have done a Reiki treatment, but it works in any situation, whether or not you have been attuned to Reiki. It clears all kinds of energy, including other people's physical sensations and emotions. It's also wonderful at helping you let go of your own stuck energy and emotions.

- Take a deep breath and fill your body with light, imagining that it is coming in through the crown of your head. You are using the Universal Life Force energy of Reiki to fill yourself. Breathe the light into your heart.

- Feel your feet on the ground and feel your connection to the ground. Push your feet into the ground. You can imagine that roots are extending from the soles of your feet into the earth.

- On the exhale breath, release any energy you picked up from the other person as if you were flushing it down the root into the earth.

- You can direct your inhale breath and the light to the part of your body that is holding the sensation and emotion.

- Do this until you no longer feel the sensations or emotions from the other person.

Emotional Empathy

With emotional empathy, we are picking up people's emotions, rather than their physical sensations. Emotional empathy is not just noticing that someone is *having* a feeling and caring that this person is having the feeling—that's sympathy. With empathy, you feel the feeling as if it was *your* feeling. For instance, imagine you're sitting next to someone who's really feeling sad. You can look at the person and notice that he or she is sad. You can feel concern about the feeling. Empaths will feel sad, too, as if the feeling originates inside of them. In energetic terms, empaths literally run someone else's emotional energy through their own system.

The first time I really noticed this was a life-changing moment for me. I was about seventeen years old and had gone to a party. I was in a great mood and happy when I went, and then I sat next to a young man who was having a really bad day and was very depressed. I listened to his story, and after about five minutes I felt sick and so upset that I started to cry. I felt horribly bad, and it had come out of nowhere! I had to leave the party. I got up and walked out, and as I left the house, I turned around and saw the young man through the window. I felt much better, like my normal self again. In that moment, I realized that it wasn't *my* feelings that I'd been feeling in there, it had been *his* feelings; I had just been feeling them right along with him!

There are two factors that can make both physical and emotional empathy very strong. One of them is *physical proximity*. You can get a big dose of what others are feeling if you're in close physical proximity to them. Maybe it's the person you're sitting next to on the airplane or at the movies, or just someone rubbing elbows with you at a party. Touching them will make it much, much stronger. With physical proximity, it doesn't matter if you know the other people or not! They could be strangers, and you will absorb whatever is going on with them.

The other factor that spurs empathy is *emotional proximity*. The closer we are to someone emotionally (best friends, family members, significant others), the more easily we can tune in to them empathically, even if they're far away from us physically. You might notice that you suddenly think of others you are close to emotionally, even if they're far away. They will hit your psychic radar because they're having a really bad day or a big emotional experience and you're tuning in long distance. When this happens, don't forget to practice the Reiki Waterfall Exercise. In fact, it's a good habit to do that exercise daily. I do it regularly before I go to bed to clear my system before I sleep. I also do it briefly between each of my clients in my Reiki practice.

Empathic Energy Transfer

As I mentioned at the beginning of this section, empaths can heal other people unconsciously, in a move called an *energy transfer*. It happens when an empath pulls someone else's energy into their own system. Let's say you're a massage therapist and you're working on someone who is having a bad day. Maybe the person is very sad and has a headache to boot. You put your hands on the person and you *feel* all that stuff. You feel bad for the person, too, and you want to help. You unconsciously absorb all his or her physical and emotional pain. You can't help it; you just "suck it up" without even knowing that you're doing it. Because your energy field is so porous, it's as easy as breathing.

The problem is that when you do this for others, not only do you absorb their energy, but you also *give* them a bunch of your own healthy energy. And, they will feel better! You sucked up all their emotional and physical pain and gave them some of your higher-frequency energy. You have basically just swapped energy with them, which is why this is called an energy transfer.

Because energy doesn't exist in a vacuum, as you give your own energy away, you leave an empty spot in your energy reserve, and your client's energy backwashes in to fill it. This is why you would walk away from that massage session feeling horrible while your client feels great! And, it all happened without you even knowing that you were doing it. Now you're stuck with whatever yucky energy the other person had and your own life-force energy is depleted.

In this kind of encounter, whoever has the lower energy wins and walks away feeling wonderful, while the person who donated higher-vibration life-force energy will feel terrible. This will also happen to an empath who is on the massage table getting a massage if the massage therapist is the one having a low-energy day.

If you don't know how to clear out the bad energy you've just collected (or you don't take the time to do so), it will accumulate, and over time it will cause a host of problems. These problems will live in your body as pain and fatigue, and in your emotions as depression and anxiety. They were not your problems to begin with, but they are now! If you swap energy with everyone you encounter throughout the day, you can see how over time an empath can end up with chronic energy depletion leading to health problems and to depression.

You can have the same kind of energy transfer happen just by listening to someone, even over the phone. That explains why some people seem to suck the life out of you even if you just casually chat with them or sit in the same room. Are you getting the picture of how totally crucial energy management is for empaths? Are you ready for some good news?

The good news is that you do not have to build your life around preventing energy loss. This is what many overwhelmed and unskilled empaths are doing when they withdraw from the world. If you do Reiki, instead of this unconscious energy transfer, you'll never have the problems of energy depletion. While your own energy and other peoples' energy flows out and in and back and forth, Reiki energy is like water flowing out of a faucet. When the water is flowing out, nothing flows back in. Because Reiki energy comes from the inexhaustible supply of universal life-force energy, you are not giving away your own energy to heal others' hurts. You can't give your own energy away when Reiki energy is flowing through you, nor can you take in the dark, wounded energy from the other person. Reiki saves the day!

Learning Reiki Level 1 is the subject of the next chapter, but before we get there, I want to teach you the grounding, clearing, replenishment, and boundary-setting skills that will keep you empowered and safe while you practice Reiki.

Basic Grounding Practices

Grounding is one those terms that gets tossed around a lot, but what does it *mean*? It means to be fully present in every way possible.

When we are grounded, we are fully present inside our own bodies and in the moment with our thoughts, and we are connected energetically to the earth. Almost everyone needs to work on this. The more empathic you are, the more you will have to practice.

The goal is to be completely present and grounded the whole time that we are doing a Reiki session. The best healing happens when you are solidly grounded and fully present, with your complete awareness focused on your client in the present moment. Then you can open your heart to compassion. When you can be wholly open and present, the modality that you're using is just the delivery mechanism for the universal love and compassion that flows through you. All healers in any modality need to learn this. When you are grounded and fully present, and your heart is open with compassion, you will transmute the suffering of your client. These are the basic ingredients for all healing, no matter what your modality is.

It's not safe for you or your client to do Reiki if you're checked out, dissociated, or not present. You wouldn't feel safe working with a therapist or doctor who was totally checked out and dissociated during your appointment, would you? When you're grounded and heart-opened, you make it safe for your clients to open up and go deep in their process. Your clients will all unconsciously feel you out to see how grounded, safe, and open you really are. They will modify how deeply they will let themselves go, and they will only release if they feel you hold a safe and sacred space for them. We call this *presence*, and being grounded is a vital part of it.

This is the real reason why some healers have a long line of clients at their door waiting to see them, and other healers are twiddling their thumbs with no clients at all. Healers with presence have clients galore. Learning presence takes practice. Sometimes it makes my heart ache to stay fully present to the suffering of another person, but I also know that it is necessary. Because I've had a lot of practice doing this, I have learned some great techniques for holding sacred space.

Here is a basic, universally applicable grounding practice. Do this at least once a day or as needed. It's very beneficial to do this after you have had an emotional upset, been somewhere with chaotic energy, or had a challenging day. Practicing it at least once a day will help make it a habit to be more grounded.

BASIC GROUNDING PRACTICE

- Push your feet into the floor and press your spine into the back of your chair

- Feel the long bones of your legs and spine.

- Breathe light into the top of your head, filling yourself up with light.

- Draw this light into your heart and belly, then exhale it down your legs and feet, and then into the earth to ground yourself.

- Now open your heart wide. Imagine it opening so big that you could fit that person and his or her trauma right inside it. Keep your eyes open and on your client. Closing your eyes can make you feel less grounded.

- Keep breathing. Breathe in the light and ground it again. Exhale out compassion.

Connecting to the Earth: The Hara Line

Now, let's talk a little about energy anatomy to help you understand more about how grounding works and how to stay grounded. The hara line is an energetic connection each of us has with the earth. Imagine a line of energy that starts at your soul and goes into the top of your head, down your spinal column, down your legs, and into the ground, continuing right down into the center of the earth. Your soul is in a dimension somewhere above the earth. Some call it "heaven," but when I was a child, I always called it "soul world." *Hara* is the Japanese word for this energy line; it is also called *shashumna* in Sanskrit, or, sometimes, the "life purpose line" in other languages and traditions.

The hara line is the central current of energy running through out bodies. The wider your hara line is, the more energy and vitality you have. Our chakras plug into the hara line, in the front and the back. When we receive a Reiki attunement, it opens and strengthens the hara line. The hara line constantly downloads energy and

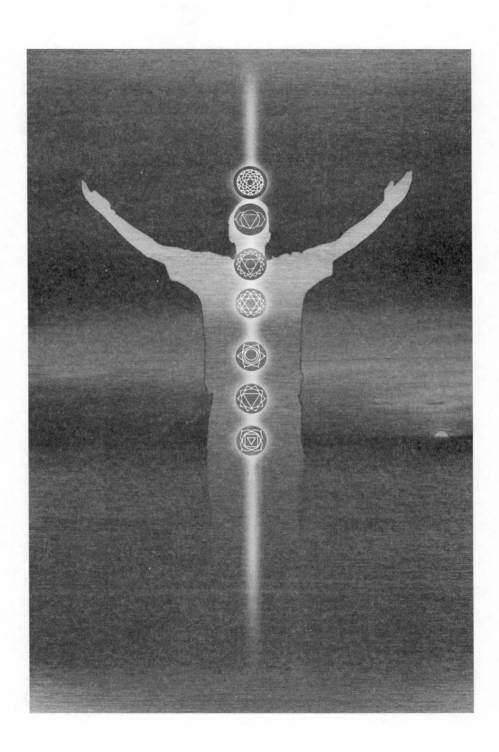

information from our souls, bringing it down to us here on earth. Pulses of energy come down this cord. We feel these pulses as moments of inspiration or intuition, or as *aha* moments.

Strengthening the Grounding Cord

The *grounding cord* is the part of the hara line that goes from the base of your spine, down your legs through the soles of your feet, to the center of the earth. It's very good to concentrate on this part of your energy system while you're doing Reiki, since it's what will keep you grounded. You can also keep your system clear of unwanted energy by flushing it down through the grounding cord.

You need to practice three things to make yourself more grounded:

1. Being in your body.

2. Being in the here and now in your thoughts.

3. Being connected to the ground through the grounding cord.

Most people have a bad energetic habit of being *out* of their bodies. Psychologists call this state *dissociation*. It takes practice and diligence to change our habit of being ungrounded. Do it by practicing your connection to your grounding cord.

CONNECTING TO THE GROUNDING CORD

-   Begin by sitting or standing up straight with your arms and legs uncrossed and your feet on the ground.

-   Take a deep breath and concentrate on your tailbone, bringing your breath right to that point.

-   As you exhale, imagine the grounding cord as a big tree root or a beam of light that extends from the base of your spine down into the ground.

- On your exhale, move the energy down your legs and out the soles of your feet.

- With each inhale breath, breathe light into the top of your head all the way down your spine to its base.

- With each exhale, imagine the grounding cord going deeper and deeper into the earth.

- Try spreading these roots out wide all round you, as well as going deep. You can make the grounding cord as wide and deep as you need it.

Repeat this practice daily, especially when you feel like you need extra grounding. Over time, it will increase your baseline grounding.

You can (and should) strengthen your grounding whenever possible. Here are some practices you can work into everyday life. Sometimes we need something other than a visualization and a breathing exercise.

Do them often, and you will reap the benefit of being as grounded as possible.

- Take your shoes off and rub your feet on the ground. Be barefoot on the ground outside as often as you can be.

- Lie with your back on the ground and breathe deeply. Feel where your spine contacts the ground. Breathe yourself into your spine by concentrating on your backbone as you breathe in.

- Rub the palms of your hands and the soles of your feet together.

- Be in nature and in contact with the earth as much as possible. Go for a walk in the woods and sit under a tree. (Or hug one!) Sit on a rock or in the grass.

- Eat something fresh or drink spring water.

- Do something ordinary: have a cup of tea, do some yard work, sweep the floor, and so forth.

- Walk briskly, stretch, or do some yoga. Exercise always brings us back into our bodies.

- Try a grounding/earthing mat. I have one under my desk when I am on the computer and one under my Reiki table for healings.

Basic Clearing Practices

Clearing is the second kind of energy management technique all healers, especially all sensitive empaths, should practice and know. *Clearing* means releasing energy that you picked up from other people. As we discussed, when you are empathic and sensitive you can pick up energy and emotions from other people just by being out and about in the world. We also pick up residual energy from our loved ones and the people we do energy work on. This is called *contact negativity*, and it is just a part of being in the world. When you drive your car around, it's going to get dirty. The same goes for our energy. It can look like a dirty brown haze on the very outer edges of the energy field, like soot, especially when we have spent time in negative or chaotic environments. Spending the day in the court-house doing jury duty and visiting a friend at the hospital are exam-ples of time spent in challenging environments for sensitives. A *chaotic* is an environment filled with lots of people, like a shopping mall, movie theater, or airport. We also have to clear to release our own energy and feelings, so we can show up with full presence to our Reiki sessions.

In addition to the breathing meditation, here are some clearing techniques that are very effective. Find a few that work for you and do them with diligence.

- Wash your hands after your Reiki session and imagine that whatever you picked up is washing down the drain.

- Imagine you're soaking your hands in a bucket of cool water. (This is very good right after a Reiki session if you can't get the heat out of your hands.)

- Imagine that you're breathing healthy, healing energy up from the ground and blowing the stale energy out through the top of your head or out of your mouth on the exhale.

- Imagine that a golden hoop goes over your head and down to your toes. Visualize that everywhere it touches, it takes negative energy out and replaces it with light. When it touches the ground, let the ground reabsorb it. (You can also go from the ground up to the sky.)

- Take a bath with sea salt or Epsom salts. Lavender and rosemary are good herbs to clear energy. You can add them right to your bathwater.

- Take a shower and imagine that the water is also clearing any negative energy with it.

- *Smudge* yourself by burning sage or incense. Clear your Reiki space often using this method. You can also use sage spray. I use sage spray on each client, the room, and myself at the end of a Reiki session.

- Kneel on the ground and then slowly lower your forehead to the ground in "child's pose" from yoga. (This is great for *emptying* out the heart and clearing the third eye.)

- Spend time in nature. Fresh air and sunlight are highly beneficial. It's best if you can get into the woods.

- Exercise—any kind is good. Breathing and sweating are great ways to clear yourself.

- Sit in a sauna or steam room.

- Meditate and engage in other spiritual practices.

- Give or receive some Reiki!

Replenishment

Many of the practices listed above in the grounding and clearing sections are also effective for the third kind of energy management: replenishment. Because of the porous nature of the empath's energy field, there is a tendency to lose energy, causing fatigue. Therefore, learning how to replace this lost energy is a key energy management technique.

To recover and replenish your energy, do anything that feeds your soul. Try exercising, being in nature, massage, Reiki, sunlight, or contact with animals or plants. Make it a point to do replenishing things every day, especially during times when lots of energy is pouring out of you. Creative pursuits like art, dancing, and music are also very replenishing.

The following exercise is a powerful and fun meditation for clearing your energy field and replenishing your energy reserves very quickly. It's called Up-and-Down Breathing, and I do it between clients if I'm seeing them back-to-back. It's wonderful if you are feeling tired: try it instead of that extra cup of coffee! It is also very effective for clearing negative or stuck energy from your energy field.

UP-AND-DOWN BREATHING

1. You can either sit or stand for this, but having your feet on the floor is important. Breathe light in through the top of your head and fill yourself with this light.

2. On the exhale breath, drop the grounding cord down. Push your feet into the floor and make sure your spine is straight.

3. Do two or three clearing breaths down the grounding cord. Release and clear on the exhale breath.

4. Next, breathe in through the top of your head and up the grounding cord at the same time, like you are sucking the energy through a straw. Take a very deep breath here. Concentrate on collecting the energy right at the solar plexus, which is the third chakra.

5. Hold your breath for a second and imagine a golden ball of energy forming at the solar plexus.

6. Exhale vigorously and imagine the golden ball moving three dimensionally out through your energy field. As this energy moves through you, it knocks off anything that is hanging on the outside of your field. It can take some practice to get this moving three dimensionally, so don't forget to imagine it behind you, above your head, and under your feet.

7. Repeat this breath five or six times. You should feel very energized, charged, and clear.

The Takeaway

The more sensitive and empathic you are, the more you will benefit from making energy management fundamentals a regular part of your life. Even if you never practice Reiki, incorporating these principles and practices into your life can help transform your relationship with the world by allowing you to keep more of your energy within yourself rather than helplessly losing it to others. It'll make you not only safer in your life, but empowered as an empath. Your gift is one that can help heal the world, and so I hope you embrace it!

In the following chapters, you are also going to learn the art of psychic protection, or shielding, which is also a critical skill that all Reiki practitioners need to learn and will be of interest to empaths. This is how we manage dark or even dangerous energy when it comes in a healing session and as we encounter it in the world. If you have an empathic child or teen, this material can be very helpful for showing you how best to parent your kid. If you are an empath, and have empathic children, learning how to manage your empathy yourself and then modeling and teaching your children what you know is a wonderful thing to do.

These practices are helpful for healers of all kinds, not just Reiki practitioners. As you practice them regularly, your energy field will become more healthy, strong, and robust, which will help you feel better able to step into your life's purpose as a healer.

In the next chapter, I will discuss the practical aspects of how to do Reiki on yourself and someone sitting in a chair. You will learn hand positions for self-healing techniques and the hand positions for "Kitchen Table Reiki." This is what I call those times when we feel called to give some Reiki during our everyday lives. We don't always need to put someone on a massage table in our office. You might want to do Reiki on a friend who comes over to your house and is in distress about something. I have done many impromptu Reiki sessions at my own kitchen table, which is how I coined the term. It's a very easy and natural way to use Reiki, and I am sure you will do a lot of Reiki this way, too.

Let's jump into the joys of Reiki Level 1!

CHAPTER 5

Reiki Level 1

In this chapter, you're going to learn the fundamentals of practicing Reiki Level 1. We will start with the mechanics of the attunement process and then move on to how to use Reiki on yourself or your friends and family—including children and pets. Every level of Reiki affects the mind, body, and spirit, but each level also has a specialty. Reiki Level 1 is focused on the body and physical healing. Often, when people get the Reiki Level 1 attunement, physical issues that have been lurking in the background will come to the forefront. Physical healings that are almost miraculous can take place with Reiki Level 1.

We are going to build a basic understanding of the hand positions to use on others and ourselves. We need to practice on ourselves first and then on other people. You'll learn in this chapter that practicing the basics will help you grow as a healer. Take your time working your way through this chapter. Pay attention to yourself and the people you give Reiki to, and how the energy moves within and between you. This is what Reiki Level 1 is all about. It's your practical foundation. Let's get started!

Reiki Level 1 Attunement

The attunement is the process by which the teacher passes the ability to do Reiki to the student. It takes about two minutes, feels great, and is a very powerful healing. You can only receive an attunement from someone who is a Reiki Master. Attunements can be done long distance. The traditional Japanese word for an attunement is *reiju*, which means "initiation." It is an initiation into the world of Reiki healing.

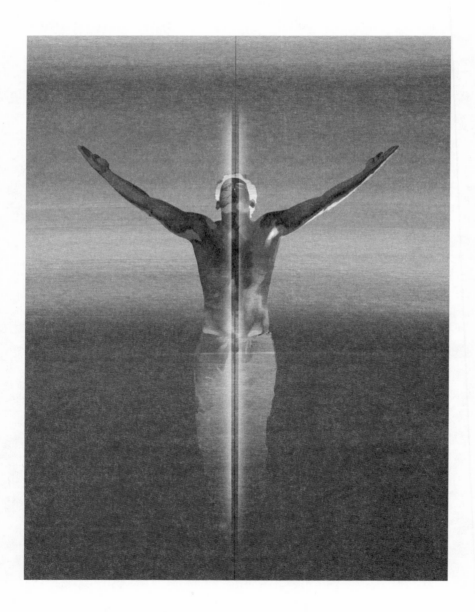

If you already have a Reiki teacher, I want to take a minute to honor your teacher. Showing honor to your teachers is an important part of Reiki. If you don't already have a Reiki teacher, you will need to find one so that you can receive a Reiki attunement. Many people meet their Reiki teachers at Reiki shares, or you might choose to work with a person who has been giving you Reiki sessions. (Reiki shares are groups of students who practice together, usually with a teacher present to give instructions.) Find someone whom you like, respect, and resonate with, since it's an important process.

The attunement works by changing your energy field in a permanent way. It allows you to flow more energy through your whole system and connects you to the frequency of Reiki. The attunement opens the crown energy center and the hara line. When you receive an attunement, the size and strength of your hara line increase. The most basic attunements open the hara line and implant the symbols into the crown energy center and palms of the hands. During the attunement, the Reiki symbols are implanted into the seventh chakra, opening the crown energy center and connecting us to Universal Life Force energy and the Reiki frequency. Once the symbols are implanted in the crown energy center, they stay there permanently.

Next, the symbols are pressed into the energy centers in the palms of the hands. Everyone has these energy centers, but they are not open on everyone. This opening allows the student to flow energy from the palms of the hands and creates the *hot hands* sensation that is so characteristic of Reiki.

Opening the crown chakra and the chakras in the palms is the most basic way to do an attunement. When I do an attunement, I also open and clear the heart chakra, implanting the symbols there as well. I do this right after I open the crown chakra and before I open the palms. Reiki is the frequency of unconditional love, so it's much more powerful and effective if the heart is clear and open. This part of the attunement connects the crown and heart center, which is how we feel unconditional love.

The final step that I do is opening and implanting the symbols in the feet, which creates more permanent grounding in the student. I found that my students could be very spacey after an attunement, so extra grounding is a good thing. There are many possible variations to the attunement process and many ways Reiki Masters attune their students. Reiki Masters attune their students as they were attuned by their masters; yours will do the same.

During the attunement, Reiki clears any damage to the student's aura and strengthens the student's energy field. Holes are repaired, chakras are cleared, and the entire energy field changes its frequency to a higher vibration. As you can imagine, attunements are very healing. It's very beneficial to get attuned frequently, even though it's not technically necessary. Once you are attuned, you are permanently connected to Reiki.

Attunement Aftereffects

The Reiki Level 1 attunement affects people in different ways. Some people don't notice a big change right away, but sometimes the effects are dramatic. Reiki attunements will make you very thirsty, so it's important to drink a lot of water right after an attunement. The Reiki Level 1 attunement increases your baseline energy frequency, which means that anything that does not resonate with this new frequency is going to leave your system. You may get nasal discharge and other cold-like symptoms, or you may have increased bowel activity or urination as your body rids itself of toxins. This is normal, and while it may be uncomfortable, it will pass. The more toxic your system is, the more likely you are to have these kinds of symptoms. If you smoke, do recreational drugs, are a heavy drinker, and eat unhealthy food, you're likely to experience some physical detox symptoms. If you live a very clean life, eat well, and exercise, you will probably have minimal physical detox effects. Drink lots of water and rest. You can also give yourself plenty of Reiki!

Now that you are attuned, you can start experiencing what it's like to heal yourself with Reiki. Some people experience an emotional reaction after their attunement. You might feel over-emotional—a little weepy, angry, or irritated. This is good, even though it doesn't feel great: releasing stuck emotions is an important part of your healing. Whatever comes up for you emotionally will be something that you're ready to let go of. It's often whatever emotion you have been blocking or denying. Again, this is natural and part of the process. If you're uncomfortable with the emotions that arise, or need help processing them, try journaling, resting, eating well, talking to a friend or a counselor, or giving yourself as much Reiki as you like. If you feel very overwhelmed and need help, talk to your Reiki teacher and seek counseling.

CAN I DO REIKI EVEN IF I'VE NEVER BEEN ATTUNED?

Natural healers have an ability to pass on their own energy to other people. Although some people spontaneously learn to use healing energy, it isn't Reiki unless you get an attunement. You want to be careful about healings in which you pass your own energy to someone else. This is an energy transfer and can negatively affect the healer. It may also not be the best thing for the person receiving the energy. As we discussed in chapter 4, there is usually a *backwash* effect, meaning the healer picks up some of the recipient's energy and whatever problems the recipient has. In this scenario, whoever has the highest frequency will feel worse since it is basically an energy swap.

Reiki insulates you from this effect, since it's not your own energy you're transferring. Reiki practitioners let the limitless, Universal Life Force energy of Reiki energy flow through them. Since Reiki energy comes from an inexhaustible source, the healer doesn't have to feel drained at the end of the session. And, the healer is also getting Reiki while doing a healing. Therefore, the Reiki healer will often feel better, more energized, and relaxed after doing a session.

Practicing Reiki After Your Level 1 Attunement

Practicing Reiki after you receive your attunement is very important. You want to give as much Reiki as you can in the days and weeks following your attunement, especially on yourself. Frequent practice makes your Reiki stronger, and it also teaches you about what Reiki feels like in your own physical and energy bodies.

A Reiki healing follows these basic steps:

- Ask permission from your recipient.

- Do Reiki breathing to ground and center yourself.

- Activate Reiki energy

- Give spot healing on a chakra or body part that needs it, or use a healing pattern by placing your hands in sequence down the recipient's energy body from head to foot.

- Turn Reiki off and step away.

- Ground and clear as you learned in chapter 4.

This basic structure works in all situations, whether you are giving yourself or someone else a bit of Reiki in the moment, sitting in a chair, or offering a full healing session on a table. Practicing it a lot in the first days and weeks after your attunement gives you two advantages:

1. Giving Reiki in a safe, structured, and respectful manner will become second nature to you.

2. You'll get your Reiki healing off to a strong start right away.

Also, as we discussed in the previous chapter, if you have strong empathic or other psychic gifts, having good habitual practices around grounding, clearing, and replenishing your energy will protect you and allow you to use those gifts powerfully in your healing work.

REIKI ON, REIKI OFF

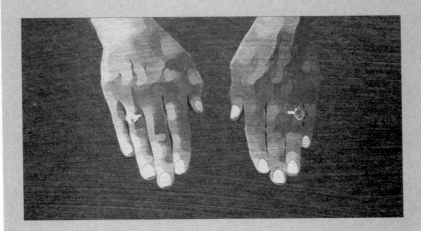

To begin a Reiki healing, we need to turn the flow of Reiki on. To do this, hold out your hands with the fingers and thumbs tucked in and say, either out loud or in your head, "Reiki on!" It's a command that assertively sets your intention. At the end of the session, do the same thing, but this time say, "Reiki off!" It's good for beginners to clearly set their intentions. In the higher levels of Reiki, it's not necessary to do this; your mental intention to begin and end a session will be sufficient, especially if you've practiced it consistently at Reiki Level 1.

This technique is useful if you're a person whose hands get very hot while doing Reiki, and the heat just won't drain from your hands. Sometimes very empathic people's hands will heat up when they're in the presence of someone who isn't feeling well, and practicing "Reiki on!" and "Reiki off!" will help you control this sensation.

Practicing Reiki Level 1 for Self-Healing

Practice makes perfect! The best way to learn Reiki is to practice as much as you can. At Reiki Level 1, the best person to practice on is yourself. Doing self-healing work will strengthen your Reiki and help support you in all areas of your life. I believe that the people with the strongest Reiki are the ones who are frequently doing self-healing as part of their Reiki practice.

Since practicing self-healing has so many advantages, it's a good idea to do a little every day. Any time you can get even one hand on yourself, you can do some self-healing. You can do Reiki on yourself while you're watching TV, driving, or falling asleep. Sitting in a boring meeting? Do some Reiki on yourself!

Ready to give it a try? Use the simple self-healing practice below to use Reiki for the first time.

SIMPLE REIKI SELF-HEALING

Sitting in a chair is the best way to do self-healing, but it can also be done while lying in bed. Begin by doing Reiki breathing and setting your intention to "Reiki on." Choose one or more of the following hand positions for self-healing. (You'll learn more about what I mean by "sandwich position" and "bridge position" in the pages that follow.) If you do a sequence of positions, move from the top of your body downward. You can try putting your hands in contact with your body, or experiment with hovering your hands over your physical body since they will still be touching your energy body. When you finish, remember to end with "Reiki off" and clear.

- Hands on the top of your own head, hovering over the crown chakra. (This opens the crown chakra.)

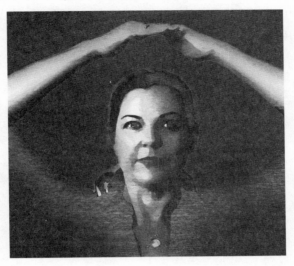

- Hands along the jawline, fingertips at the temples. (Move the energy back and forth between your palms to balance the hemispheres of the brain and calm the mind.)

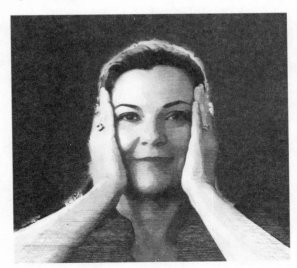

- Hands at the front and back of the forehead, in a sandwich position. (Move the energy back and forth between your palms to balance the brain from the front to the back. This will stop overthinking.)

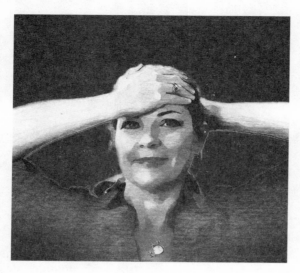

- Palms on the neck. (This position helps open up your voice, so you can say what you need to say.)

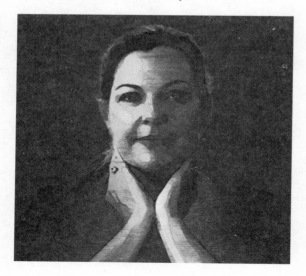

- Hands on the heart. (Opens and activates the heart and clears grief.)

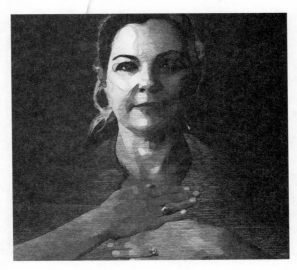

- Bridge position between the heart and solar plexus. (This is the best position for relieving anxiety.)

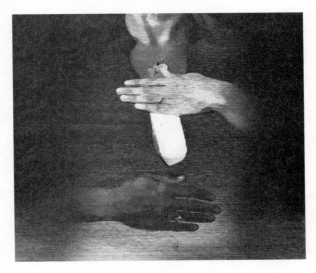

- Hands on the solar plexus. (This is good for digestive complaints.)

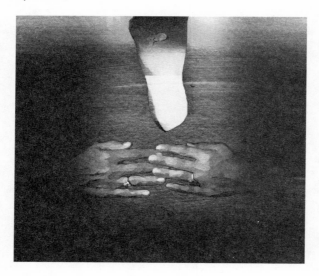

- Bridge position between the solar plexus and the navel. (This calms the emotions in general.)

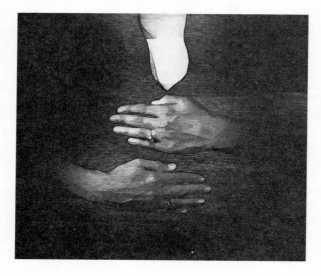

- Hands on the navel. (This is good for lower digestive complaints, lower back pain, and any reproductive issues.)

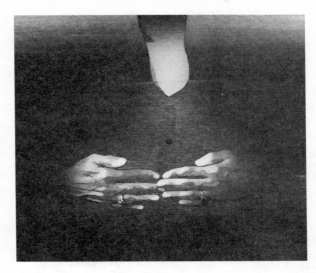

- Bridge position between the shoulders and the hands. (This is good for general tension and stress.)

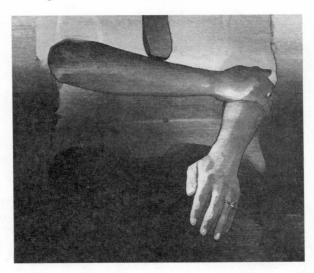

- Bridge position between the outer hip and the knee. (This position works the root chakra to help you feel more secure in life and more grounded.)

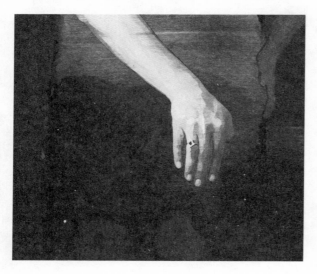

- Bridge position between the knee and the foot. (This is another excellent way to ground yourself.)

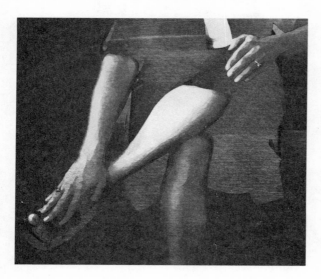

Really open your heart and flow some love your own way. I can't stress enough the power of healing yourself. Many people ask me how to love themselves more, and this is an awesome way to do it!

EXPERIMENT WITH REIKI

The first few days and weeks that you do Reiki is a special time. Use it to build good habits and pay attention to the experiences you are having with your new abilities. Every time you give Reiki to yourself or someone else, take a bit of time afterward to reflect on the experience. What was your state going into the session and during it? How did you feel afterward? What came up for you? Did you experience any psychic or intuitive hits? Did you check them with the recipient?

Write your observations in your psychic journal, and record details, such as who you gave Reiki to, when and for how long, what hand positions you used, what decisions you made based on your intuition, and what the results were for you and your recipient. Becoming adept at a healing modality takes time and practice, and your notes will become a record of your progress and a resource for deeper learning.

Paying careful attention to all your experiences as you give Reiki is essential for you as a psychically gifted person. You are developing your healing gifts and your psychic gifts and learning how to protect and care for yourself as you do it. Take your time to be mindful and loving to yourself.

Hand Positions for Reiki Level 1

In Reiki Level 1, we learn the hand positions for doing Reiki on ourselves and on others who are sitting in a chair. It's very useful to know how to work with someone who is sitting in a chair since we often won't always have a Reiki table handy. I call this "Kitchen Table Reiki." This happens when you're hanging out with someone at your kitchen table who's having a bad day. Maybe this person is suffering with a headache, stress, or an emotional upset of some kind. You end up offering Reiki, so you put your hands on the person's head and heart and do some Reiki as he or she sits in a chair. I've done many "Kitchen Table Reiki" sessions and value them just as much as the formal Reiki sessions done in my office.

In the pages that follow, I'll teach you basic Reiki Level 1 hand positions, talk through the principles you should pay attention to while you're giving Reiki, and then give you some sequences for putting the positions together in a session.

These hand positions are like a recipe. Once you learn the basic *ingredients*, you might find that your hands just *want* to go somewhere that isn't listed here, or that is listed in a different order. Go with what feels right. Those hunches, impressions, or ideas is your intuition giving you information about how to best help that person. One of the best things about Reiki is that we can so easily combine it with our intuition and psychic ability to tailor a treatment for what our recipient needs in that moment. Go with your intuition!

Sandwich Positions

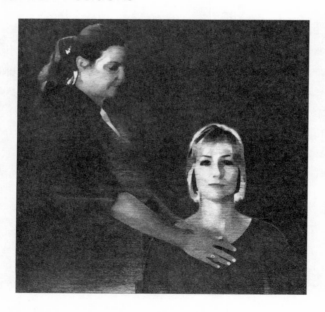

When a hand position is described as a *sandwich position*, it means that you sandwich a body part between your two hands. A *heart sandwich* is when you have one hand on the front of the heart and the other hand on the back of the heart. When you're doing a sandwich position, your goal is to move the energy back and forth between your hands so that the energy becomes balanced. Use your intention to move the energy back and forth between your palms until your hands feel balanced and the energy is moving evenly between them. This balances the energy evenly between the back and front aspects of a chakra.

Sandwich positions also work wonders for parts of the body that have physical damage. If you fall and hurt your knee, do Reiki on it with a sandwich position as soon as you can! Sandwich positions work well for smaller parts of the body, too. You can pretty much cover the whole foot, for example, if you do a foot sandwich.

Sandwich positions are the best for:

- Filling up depleted chakras

- Clearing blocked chakras

- Relieving pain and bringing healing to a specific area

- Handling an emotional upset (heart sandwich)

Bridge Positions

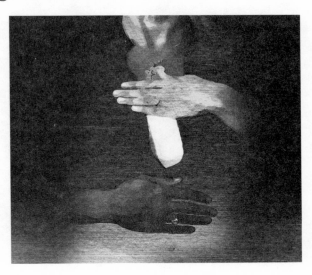

A *bridge position* is when you put one hand on one chakra and the other hand on another chakra to connect them. When you connect two different parts of the body (for example, one hand on the heart and the other on the solar plexus), it creates an energy flow between the two chakras and balances them.

Using bridge positions brings balance to the whole system, especially the central nervous system, and creates deep relaxation in the body.

- The crown and brow bridge calms and settles the mind.

- The throat and heart bridge helps you talk about your feelings.

- The heart and solar plexus bridge relieves anxiety.

- The heart and navel bridge calms down emotions in general.

- The navel and root bridge (one hand on the belly, the other on the knees) helps ground your emotions.

Spread Positions

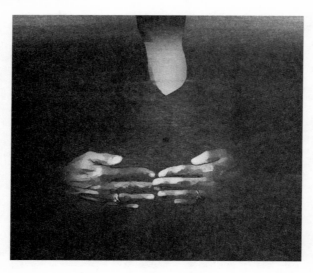

A *spread position* is when you spread your hands out across the body, rather than in the midline of the body. When you're working down the midline of the body, you're working on a chakra. With a spread position, you're working on the organs and tissues of the body itself, rather than a chakra.

For example, the third chakra is right in the solar plexus. If you put both hands on the solar plexus, you're working on the chakra. But if you spread your hands out across the ribs, you're sending Reiki to the organs of the body that are located here, specifically the liver, gallbladder, spleen, and stomach.

Sometimes we need to direct energy to the chakra, and other times we need to send it to the body itself. This chakra is about personal power, your will, and your self-esteem. If you want to clear a block around someone's self-esteem, you would send Reiki into this chakra. This chakra also rules our metabolism and, therefore, all digestive organs.

If your recipient is having a problem with her gallbladder, you would use a spread position to work on the organ itself. Of course, the two are very likely connected. Suffering from poor self-esteem for a long time will block this chakra, creating a negative impact on the organs of the third chakra.

Each of the organs holds an emotional and spiritual meaning. For example, the gallbladder holds the energy of resentment and bitterness. If your recipient doesn't love herself enough to set good boundaries in her life and overgives and then feels resentful when no one gives back, she's going to have gallbladder problems eventually.

Principles for Giving Reiki

There are a few basic principles for giving Reiki, no matter what the level. These are good, general guidelines to follow as you are giving your Reiki treatments.

Work from the Top Down

Start at the head and work all the major parts of the body, working your way down to the toes. In some modalities, you work from the feet up toward the head, but in Reiki we always work from the head down.

If someone is bothered by something very specific—a headache, an emotional upset, or an injury—it's fine to just treat the one affected area. This is called *spot treating*. Or, if you only have a few minutes, just do the head, shoulders, and heart areas. If you fall and hurt your knee, you can just work on your knee. No need to work all the way down your body from your head to get to it.

Working On and Off the Body

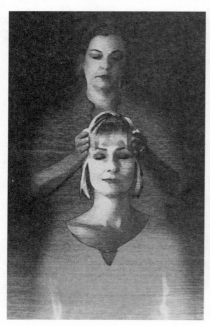
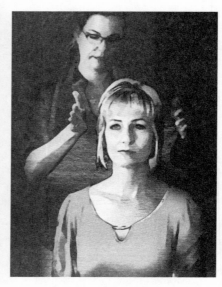

Some people aren't comfortable being touched, so it's important to know how to work off the body if you need to. You can do a whole Reiki session without ever touching your recipient. Reiki works just as well when you hover your hands a few inches off the body. When you do this, you're still working inside their energy field. Some Reiki practitioners *only* work off the body.

I'm a pretty touchy-feely person and prefer to work hands-on. I feel that people really benefit from healthy, nonsexual, nurturing touch. It's a deep human need, and most people don't get enough of it. Therapeutic touch can be very nurturing and healing, so I prefer to work hands-on when I can—always with the client's permission.

Ask Permission

It's very important to ask permission to give Reiki to someone. For hands-off Reiki, something simple like "May I give you some Reiki?" works fine. If you wish to add hands-on work, make sure you ask permission each time. "Is it okay with you if I touch you, or would you rather I just work off your body?" I start every Reiki session that I do by asking my recipient, "Are you comfortable being touched?"

Not everyone likes to be touched, and it's within everyone's right to refuse it, including children. It's so important to *always* get permission. Doing "stealth" Reiki without asking for permission is a violation of people's free will, even if you think you are doing it for their own good and have the best intentions.

Work with Your Eyes Open

It's very important when you're doing Reiki to work with your eyes open. So many Reiki practitioners work with their eyes shut during their sessions. I don't recommend this. You need to stay in visual contact with your recipient throughout your entire interaction. It's much more grounding for the practitioner. If you're a person who has trouble staying grounded while you're doing Reiki, keep your eyes open. Also, you'll have no idea what is happening with your recipient if your eyes are shut. If your recipient cries, has an energetic release, or goes into distress, you'll want to be aware of that.

I went to a Reiki share once, where everyone was working with eyes closed. One poor lady on the table was in clear distress—crying, twitching, and generally freaking out. Her practitioner was totally unaware of this because her eyes were shut tight and she was probably communing with her angels. She was having a grand old time and was very clearly checked out. She finally opened her eyes when the recipient started gagging and was shocked to find that things weren't going so well for her recipient.

I've also seen a Reiki practitioner with eyes shut feeling around on the recipient, looking for the next hand position. There was some very inappropriate, if unintentional, touching happening. I was horrified (as was the recipient) watching as this practitioner groped at the recipient's chest, trying to find her heart chakra and getting a handful of something else.

Work with your eyes open; you need to be present for your recipient. This is especially true while you're learning Reiki Level 1. As you progress through the levels, there will be times when you *can* shut your eyes for brief periods of time—while checking in with your intuition, for instance. But, then it's good to open them again.

Breathe!

Reiki flows with our breath, so make sure you are breathing a lot while you are giving Reiki. Long, slow breathing patterns work the best. Try out the "ocean breath" from the yoga tradition, which is a four-count inhale and a four-count exhale that initiates from deep in the belly. If energy feels stuck somewhere, deepening your own breath can help tremendously. If you notice recipients holding their breath, remind them to breath too. I notice that if I suddenly hold my breath, chances are good my client is also doing that, and it's my physical empathy showing me that.

We learn as children to hold our breath when we want to avoid feeling and expressing emotions. For example, you might hold your breath to prevent yourself from crying. Breathing will move energy and release emotions, so make sure both you and your recipient are breathing deeply.

Feeling Energy While You Are Doing Reiki

Not everyone can feel Reiki energy, but that doesn't mean that it's not flowing. Some people have a natural capacity to feel and sense energy flowing through them, while other people don't. The great thing about Reiki is that you don't *have* to feel it for it to work.

If you are receiving Reiki, you might feel heat, tingling, pulsing, or a wavelike sensation. Some people feel coolness rather than heat or a sensation of pins and needles, and some don't feel anything at all. If you don't feel any Reiki flowing at a certain spot, it might be because that spot is already *full*, and you should try another one. The most important thing is to be confident that the Reiki is working, even if your recipient doesn't feel it. (And, even if *you* don't feel it.)

I've done sessions where I didn't feel anything much, but my clients were seeing colors, or they felt waves of energy moving through them, and it was a big thing for them. I've also had sessions where I felt a lot, but my client didn't feel a thing. Both types of experiences can be part of a powerful Reiki session. Almost everyone receiving Reiki will feel the effects of the session. They leave feeling relaxed, calm, peaceful, warm, and nurtured. This is what really matters. Don't worry too much if you're not feeling much at Reiki Level 1. You'll learn to feel more and more over time and with practice.

Often, when there is a major energetic release for the client, I feel it in my own body. If you're an empath, you will too. I feel a big *whoosh* of energy releasing down my spine with a corresponding deep exhale. Remember that empaths will feel the recipient's energy release in their own body, so it's good to continually monitor what is happening in your own body as you are working.

Cold Spots

If you put your hands on someone to do Reiki and the place you touch feels cold to you, then it could mean that there's a lack of energy in that chakra, and that area needs to be filled with energy. The chakra is probably depleted, or there's a lack of life-force energy in the body tissues there. It can also mean that there's an energy *block* there, which is a place where energy gets stuck and can't flow freely.

If there's a serious depletion, it can take a long time to feel energy flowing there. It might take ten minutes before it starts to heat up or tingle. Leave your hands there until you feel heat and warmth come back to that spot. Remember, you can't make a mistake, so keep your hands there if you feel like it and see what happens. Of course, if you feel like moving on to a different spot, follow your instincts. Use your breath to help the energy flow.

When you're doing a sandwich position, you'll often feel that one side of the chakra is cold, empty, stuck, or depleted, and the other side is warm, pulsing, and tingling. When this happens, send energy back and forth between your hands until they both feel warm and flowing.

The Energy Crescendo

If your hands are on the same spot for a while and it's very stuck, you will eventually feel the energy begin to amplify. It will continue to build toward an energetic release. The energy (heat, tingling, pulsing, and so on) flows faster and stronger (hands getting hotter and hotter) until it reaches the crescendo. This feels like a dam bursting or a big release of energy. You may notice that your recipient feels this too; the person may sigh, twitch, or have a change in breathing. After the release point, the energy will drain away from your hands rather quickly. If you have enough time, it's best to keep your hands in one spot until you feel the crescendo; it's very beneficial to the recipient, as it means whatever block was there has cleared. Once the energy drains, you can move your hands. If you keep your hands in the same place, you'll get another crescendo and release in the same spot.

You'll experience the signs of energetic release in your recipient in any or all the following ways:

- A change in breathing, such as a sigh

- Twitching or other involuntary movements

- Blinking

- A physical emotional response (crying, smiling, and so forth)

- A rush of energy down the recipient's body

I always feel it as a rush of energy down my own spine along with a deep exhale, so don't forget to check in with your own body as you are doing this.

A Basic Reiki Level 1 Session

Now that you know the basics of hand positions for Reiki Level 1, and some principles to keep in mind while you're giving it, let's see what a simple session of Reiki Level 1 would look like. This is based on a session where we work from the top of the body down to the feet, with the recipient sitting in a chair.

First, you ask permission to do Reiki, finding out whether your recipient wants you to work on or off the body. Clear and ground yourself with Reiki breathing, then set your intention and turn Reiki on.

The Handshake Position (Hands on the Shoulders)

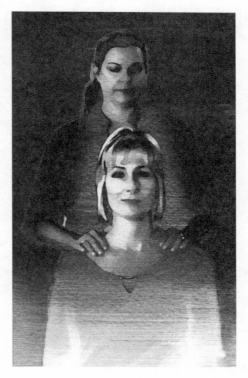

Stand behind your recipient, who is seated in a chair. Place your hands gently on the shoulders and allow her to get used to you being in her energy field. After a short amount of time, you might feel a "clicking together" feeling as your energy field begins to resonate with your recipient. This position is a gentle way to begin and end the Reiki session, as the shoulders are a neutral place to rest your hands on someone's body. It's nice to allow people to get used to us being in their energy field before we plop our hands on top of their heads!

Positions for the Head

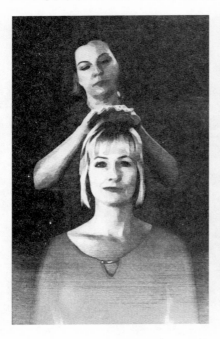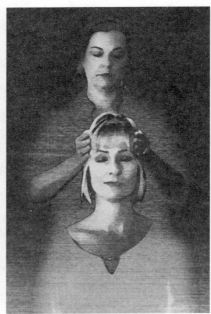

We always begin Reiki on the recipient's head and work our way down. There are a several hand positions used for working on the head.

1. Hands on the crown (top) of the head: Place your hand above the crown of the head, and allow it to hover there. It's better not to put your hands directly on the head, since this tends to close the crown chakra.

2. Hands at the sides of the head just above the ears: Use a sandwich position, one hand about an inch away from the skin on each side of the face. Move the energy back and forth between your hands to balance the hemispheres of the brain. This calms and soothes an anxious mind.

3. Hands at the forehead and occiput (back of the skull): Stand at the recipient's shoulder and, using a sandwich position, put one hand on the forehead and one on the back of the head at the occiput. Move the energy back and forth between your hands.

Throat Chakra Sandwich

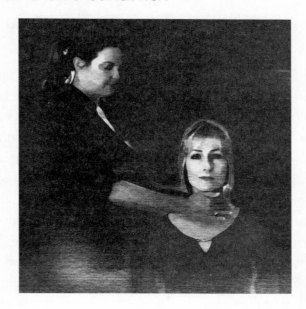

Stand at your recipient's shoulder. Put one hand at the nape of the neck and gently hover your other hand at the front of the throat. Most people don't like having their throats touched, so working off the body in a hover position is important.

Heart Chakra Sandwich

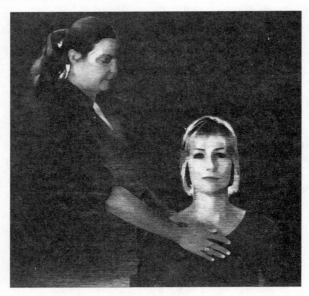

Standing at the shoulder of your recipient, put one hand at the upper chest, or over the heart, and the other hand at the back of the heart chakra, between the shoulder blades. This is also called the *heart sandwich* and is very healing. We tend to feel grief and sadness in the body at the back of the heart between the shoulder blades. We instinctively want to rub people there when they need comfort.

Most people need a lot of Reiki in the heart. We all have broken or bruised hearts, and we carry unexpressed grief about a million different things. Spend as much time as you're able to on someone's heart. Watch your hand position here. Make sure your thumb is tucked in and not jabbing the person in the throat. And make sure your hand is high up on the breastbone if you are working on a woman, and not on the breasts.

Solar Plexus Chakra

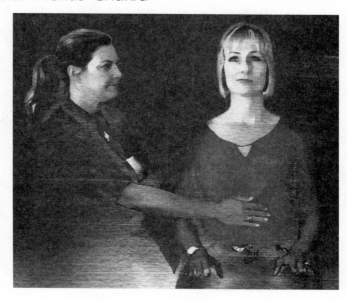

You can easily touch the back of the solar plexus, even if the recipient is sitting in a chair. (Think of where a bra strap goes across the back and you'll get the correct hand position.) Reiki will go through a chair, so you can touch the back of a chair to access this point if need be.

Hovering your hands over the front of someone's solar plexus is a good way to Reiki this spot. Many people feel uncomfortable when someone touches their belly. It's a place we tend to feel very vulnerable about, and it requires a lot of trust to let someone touch us there without raising our defenses. Also, many people have "belly shame" and are self-conscious about being touched there. Hovering over this area will help people receive energy here in a more relaxed way.

Navel Chakra Sandwich

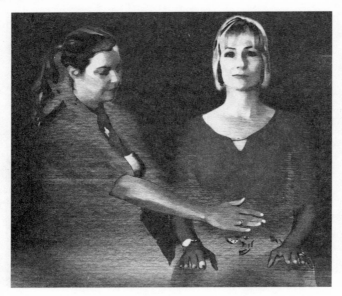

The second chakra is at the sacrum, the large, flat bone between the hips at the lower back, and many people have pain, problems, and stuck energy here since it's where emotional and sexual energy are held. We Reiki the second chakra in the same way that we Reiki the third chakra; hover low on the belly below the navel. You can touch the back of the second chakra even if the recipient is in a chair.

Bridging Shoulder to Elbow and Elbow to Hand

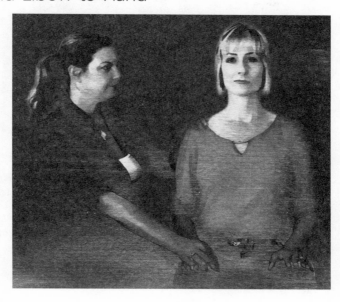

Since Reiki flows downhill, we do the arms with one hand on the shoulder and the other on either the elbow or the hand. The Reiki will flow from the top hand (shoulder hand) down. I always end with just holding the hand since there is something very comforting about having one's hand held.

It's good to pay attention to the arms and not ignore them. They are connected to the heart chakra and can become filled with unexpressed grief. Of course, the shoulders always hold a lot of tension, so releasing the energy down the arms is very relaxing.

Bridging Hips, Knees, and Feet

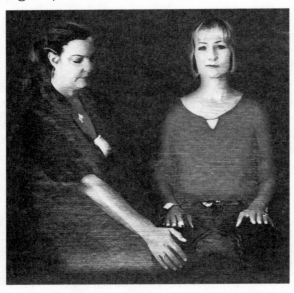

The legs are done in the same manner as the arms, starting with one hand on the outside of the hip and the other on either the knee or the foot. People often have knee or foot pain and usually need a sandwich there. Giving Reiki to the feet can help ground someone who has had a shock.

Remember to work both sides of the body. It feels weird to be left asymmetrical.

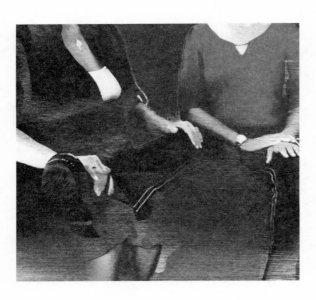

Return to Handshake Position

Finish the session by standing behind the person and going back to the handshake position, with your hands on the shoulders. Step away from the person when you're done. Do this mindfully, with the idea of energetically separating from the person. Finish with the Reiki breath, so that you can release any energy you might have picked up during your session.

The information we've discussed should give you a practical foundation for your Reiki Level 1 work. I covered how the attunement works and gave you some solid starting points, from how to begin a session to the hand positions used for someone sitting in a chair. It's best to weave in your energy management and intuitive practices along the way so that you can do Reiki without taking anything home from your recipients, too.

Self-healing is one of the best gifts of Reiki Level 1, so practice on yourself. Don't forget that the best way to make your Reiki stronger is to practice as often as you can—on your friends and family, as well as self-healing. Almost everyone wants to try it right away on their family, including their children, teens, and pets. When we are working on children, teens, and pets there are certain considerations that are different from when we are working with other adults. In the next section, I will cover the unique aspects of working on children and teens so that you can work effectively with these recipients.

Reiki Level 1 for Children and Teens

If you are a parent, you will probably want to do Reiki on your kids. Working with kids is one of the coolest things about learning Reiki Level 1. When my kids were little, they had a choice between a Band-Aid or Reiki, and most of the time they picked Reiki. It's a great tool for soothing sick children and dealing with the normal bumps and bruises, too. Reiki is a great thing to have in your medicine chest.

If your kids are very small they won't need or want much Reiki when they're feeling well and healthy. If they're feeling good, they might take Reiki for a few minutes before running away to play. But, if they're sick, they'll be docile and will enjoy a lot of Reiki.

Just a little warning: If you're dealing with stomach upset, make sure you are appropriately prepared by being in the bathroom or by having a bucket nearby before you do Reiki. If someone is going to throw up, it will happen almost immediately once you start the Reiki, so make sure you're ready for that. Too many Reiki parents find this out the hard way!

Hand Positions for Kids

When my kids were young, I did Reiki with them sitting on my lap. A really nice time to work on children is when they're falling asleep. My daughter still likes Reiki when she has a little insomnia, and she's sixteen years old. Some Reiki practitioners specialize in working with children and families, but everyone can easily work on their own kids. It's a beautiful thing to do.

Here are some hand positions and other suggestions for doing Reiki on kids:

- Spot treat. If they bump or bruise something, you can just treat that place.

- Work from the head down.

- Use your intuition. Let yourself just feel where to put your hands.

- Use your logic. If they are coughing, work on their chest.

- Kids with asthma do very well with Reiki. Work on their armpits to access the lungs.

- A little goes a long way. A full session on a small child might only take ten to twenty minutes.

- Kids with ADD benefit from one hand on each temple. Bounce the energy back and forth between your hands to balance their thinking.

- Do the heart sandwich on a crying child. (Hands on the front and back of the heart.)

- Hold the third chakra (solar plexus) on an anxious child.

- One hand on the heart and one on the head will help a child fall asleep.

Attuning Children

When my kids were little, I gave them all Reiki Level 1 attunements repeatedly. My middle son used to ask me to "tune his head," and my oldest grew up with Reiki to the point where now, as an adult, he's a Reiki Master himself.

Very young children can benefit from a Reiki Level 1 attunement, but I would wait until they're teenagers before allowing them to receive the Reiki Level 2 attunement, and I'd wait until they're close to eighteen years old before receiving the Reiki Level 3 attunement.

Children who learn Reiki don't seem to need much instruction on how to do it. I usually teach them a few hand positions to give them a general idea of how it's done. They figure out very quickly how intuitive Reiki is, and they just naturally go with the flow. It's very precious to hear them say, "Mom, you look a little tired; do you want some Reiki?"

If your kids want to be attuned at Reiki Level 1, it's a very good thing to do. Once they are attuned by a Reiki Master, you can teach them some basic self-healing hand positions, too. We're never too young to learn self-healing!

❀ Sam's Story ❀
Reiki Relief for a Psychic Child

Samantha was only eight years old when I taught her Reiki. Her grandmother brought her in because she was very psychic and was seeing "things" in the house. It was upsetting her mother and the rest of the family, too. When Sam was really little she had long conversations with dead relatives and talked to the fairies in the garden. Sam started to have anxiety problems and exhibiting

OCD-like behaviors. She had been made fun of by a friend for her psychic experiences and was now feeling bewildered and afraid of them.

Sam had powerful mediumship abilities, and like most psychic kids she was a ghost magnet. She attracted every ghost in her neighborhood, and this was making her lose sleep. I worked with Samantha, with her grandmother in the room with us. (When I work on children under the age of sixteen, I always work with a parent or guardian in the room with me, or with the door open and the parent sitting with a good line of sight to the child through the open door.)

We talked a lot about her psychic ability, and I shared experiences from my own childhood. I told her how to tell the difference between a helpful guide and an undesired presence. I showed her how to get rid of the ones that she didn't like, and I explained why the ones with the dead faces needed a lot of help, that they were stuck in their death state and needed help crossing over.

The conversation was very affirming to Sam, and she was reassured by having someone to talk to. I decided to attune her in that session, because I thought it would help her with her anxiety. She was up for it, so we spent maybe half an hour with the Reiki basics.

I saw Sam for another session a few months later, and she was doing much better. She told me that she gave Reiki to herself to help her sleep, and to her mother who was "nervous about everything." She had also figured out how to give the stuck souls some Reiki—she had learned to cross them over herself, and she thought the Reiki had really helped with that skill.

Reiki and Teens

Reiki is very empowering for teens. I have kids starting at about thirteen years old in my Reiki classes, usually with a parent or other family member. Teens often feel very disempowered in their lives in general, but especially around their emotions. Reiki can be helpful and validating for them, and it gives them a sweet way to connect not only to themselves, but to each other, too.

I do think that one should wait until kids are a little older to attune them at Reiki Level 3. Many teachers say it's good to wait until they're at least eighteen before teaching them Reiki Level 3. However, I evaluate this on a case-by-case basis, and I have chosen to give a few very mature sixteen- and seventeen-year-olds the Reiki Level 3 attunement.

I held classes and did attunements for my son and his friends when he was a teenager, and I enjoyed having teenage boys in the Reiki shares that I hosted. I would have a room full of middle-aged women and five or so teenage boys. So sweet!

One of my favorite things to do is a Reiki Level 1 mother-and-daughter class. It's always a lot of fun and a lovely bonding and sharing activity.

✿ *Robbie's Story* ✿
Healing After a Brain Injury

Robbie suffered a traumatic brain injury due to a concussion. Robbie was a football player in high school and had to stop playing because of his injury, which left him with severe anxiety and depression.

Robbie had a whole team of healers working with him, including physicians, a psychiatrist, and counselors. His mother brought him to me to help him with relaxation, since Robbie had said that the Reiki sessions worked best for managing his anxiety. He was also very psychic, and sometimes he had trouble telling what was real and what wasn't. His psychiatrist told him that his visions where hallucinations due to psychosis, but there were also times when he was sure he was seeing spirits for real.

This happens sometimes to highly psychic people. My theory is that the brain injury damaged his sixth chakra, so he was experiencing distortions in his psychic vision. It was extremely upsetting and disorienting for him. He had also had some additional trauma in his past, so his visions were negative and scary to him.

We worked together for some time as his brain injury stabilized. Eventually, Robbie's brain healed and he learned to manage his psychic gifts, too. As that happened, he learned to distinguish the difference between images of his past trauma and a real spirit visitation. After that, he was able to move into the next phase of his life on much better footing.

❀ *Emily's Story* ❀
A Young Empath in Trouble

Emily was a beautiful young woman who was so empathic and sensitive that she had trouble being in high school. The emotional overload from being at school was overwhelming to her, and she suffered from migraines, panic attacks, and depression. She missed a lot of school, even though she was an honors student, was falling behind. Emily and her mother were worried that if she couldn't get a handle on her empathy, she might jeopardize her college opportunities.

Emily needed basic training in how to manage being an empath. She was very glad to learn that there was a good reason she was empathic, and that she wasn't just crazy. She felt much better knowing that she was special, and that her gifts were meant for something good.

I recommended that she learn Reiki, and to also concentrate on the energy management basics that all empaths need to learn: ground, clear, and protect. She was the person in her social group who everyone came to talk to when they had problems, and she felt very depressed when she couldn't help them. Learning Reiki gave her a great way to help her friends. Soon, she was doing Reiki on everyone she knew and feeling much better.

The energy management basics and self-healing techniques took care of her migraines, and she was back on track. She loved Reiki so much that she went through all three levels before she went to college.

I love working with children and teens. They are so open to energy and intuitive experience and haven't become hardened in the way that many adults have. Also, I believe that they are more sensitive than adults, perhaps because they haven't yet learned to shut down their abilities. Children and teens benefit tremendously from both receiving Reiki treatments and from learning Reiki. The teens I've worked with find learning Reiki to be highly empowering in their lives. I encourage you to work with the kids and teens in your life.

The Takeaway

I hope you enjoyed your journey into Reiki Level 1. There is a lot to remember at this level when you are new to it all, but the most important thing to keep in mind about practicing Reiki is to do it with mindfulness and good awareness of what is happening in both you the practitioner and your recipient. Having good energy-management habits and keeping a tight and clean boundary will ensure your success with practicing Reiki.

All too many people step away from practicing Reiki because they don't know how to clear themselves during and after a session and walk away feeling funky. If you keep strong energetic boundaries, you will be able to move confidently to the next level of Reiki with an excellent foundation.

Reiki Level 1 is for self-healing and for working on your friends, family members, and your pets (see the Appendix by Sharon Wilsie). You can stay at this level of Reiki for as long as you feel like it. There is no need to hurry to the next level, and much can be gained by going slowly and taking in how Reiki Level 1 feels for you.

In the next chapter, we will dive into Reiki Level 2, the Practitioner's Level. You'll learn the three Reiki Level 2 symbols and how to use them, how to do Reiki on a table, and how to give Reiki long distance. I'll also help you deepen your psychic abilities and connect with your Reiki guides. This is the part of Reiki Level 2 that most people who are also psychically, intuitively, or empathically gifted find the most fascinating and fulfilling to learn.

CHAPTER 6

Reiki Level 2

Welcome to Reiki Level 2! At Reiki Level 2, you'll learn how to work with recipients more formally. After you have completed this level of training, you have enough information and experience to begin to work with clients in a professional setting. It's a good time to get an office and see clients for a fee.

Reiki Level 2 blends easily with other modalities. For example, nurses add Reiki to their nursing skills so that they are doing Reiki for their patients whenever they are touching them. It's the same for massage therapists and other body workers. If you are already a body worker, your clients will experience a huge value in adding Reiki to whatever you are doing.

In this chapter, you will learn the three Reiki Level 2 symbols. The symbols are very old and part of an ancient Japanese spiritual tradition. The symbols are used for meditation, and in healing they help to channel the Reiki energy for a specific purpose. There are symbols for physical healing, emotional healing, and mental healing.

You'll also learn about long-distance healing, which is useful when we can't put our hands on someone directly. It might be a loved one who lives far away, or the person zooming by you in an ambulance, or a group of people you see on TV who are suffering from a disaster. Or, it might be someone in the same room with you whom you can't touch for professional reasons, like a teacher and a student. With Reiki Level 2, you will also learn hand positions for someone lying on a Reiki table, rather than sitting in a chair.

Reiki Level 2 deepens psychic development. Almost everyone who receives the Reiki Level 2 attunement reports an increase in psychic insight and intuition. This is the time when you will be directly introduced to your Reiki guides. These are benevolent and helpful spiritual beings who are with us always, but especially when we are doing Reiki healing sessions. You'll learn more about Reiki guides in the next chapter.

At Reiki Level 2, many people become much more sensitive to perceiving energy during their sessions. You may begin to sense energy shifting, or start to see or feel colors. Whereas Reiki Level 1 addresses the physical level of people, Reiki Level 2 taps into the emotional level. You might notice that your recipients are more emotional on the table, or they have big emotional issues crop up. Reiki treatments can create an opportunity for someone to release an emotional issue that has been hiding in the background. When buried emotions come to a head, it's because the person is ready for it and the time is right for a healing.

We hold stuck emotional energy in our organs and muscle tissue, as well as in our chakras. We carry stuck, unresolved trauma in the nervous system and fascia/connective tissue, causing nervous system disorders. Reiki Level 2 can be very useful in clearing out and healing both unresolved emotions and unresolved traumas.

In this chapter, you will learn some techniques to help guide people through their emotional releases. It's important to learn how to do this so you will be comfortable if your client cries, for example. Recipients will unconsciously feel whether you can support their emotional release, and they will hold back from it if you can't, so it's critical that you know how to handle emotional release with comfort and ease.

True and deep healing often requires an emotional release, so as Reiki practitioners we welcome any emotions that come up for our clients.

In this chapter, you will learn:

- How to draw and use the three Reiki Level 2 symbols

- Hand positions for Reiki healing on the table, including a good basic sequence to use

- Emotional healing techniques

- Long-distance healing

The personal healing at this level can be profound and life changing, and I am excited to take you on this journey. Let's dive in now and look at what it takes to be a Reiki practitioner.

The Reiki Level 2 Symbols

At Reiki Level 1, we used "plain" Reiki, the frequency of unconditional love, flowing through us and into our recipient. At Reiki Level 2, we continue to use the three Reiki symbols—one each for physical healing, emotional healing, and mental healing—to channel and shape the flow. Adding the Reiki symbols to your toolkit expands your healing ability exponentially. As you do more healing and grow into your skills, using the symbols allows you to more precisely tailor the healing toward what the recipient needs in the moment.

There's a lot of variation among Reiki lineages about the origin of the Reiki symbols, and even their number. The original Usui Reiki School uses only four symbols. Three of them are learned at Reiki Level 2, and then the Master Symbol, which is used when giving attunements, is learned at Reiki Level 3.

The original symbols that Usui Sensei used combine traditional Japanese characters (kanji) with some influences from old Sanskrit sutras. According to Bronwen and Frans Stiene (2008), in Usui Sensei's time the symbols were given to students as something to chant about and meditate on. They were tools to help students overcome a spiritual obstacle as part of their spiritual discipline. They symbolized universal principles, such as "Align your energy with Divine energy."

If you have studied with other teachers, you may have noticed that there are many variations to each symbol. As one teacher passed them on to another, variations crept in. It's not hard to see why this might happen, since the symbols are complex. If you have learned the symbols one way and are very comfortable with them, then it's fine to stick with what you already know. The symbols have meaning, but when they are used during a Reiki healing they act more like a key to help us connect with a particular frequency. The power of the symbol comes from the connection made to that frequency during your attunement, so please use whichever versions you're most comfortable with.

The three Reiki symbols you will learn here point the main power current toward three different things:

- Physical healing

- Emotional healing

- Mental and long-distance healing

The order of these three levels is very important because it reflects the order in which people become ill. A physical problem or condition can emerge or worsen when we hold on to a stuck emotion for a long time. Stuck emotions grow from a simple thought. Perhaps you have the painful thought *I'm not worthy.* That thought feeds a feeling of shame. The feeling of shame gets lodged in the third chakra. As time goes on, this stuck feeling will create problems in the body.

For example, let's say that Susie has a gallbladder issue. Her presenting issue is pain related to gallstones. But, before there was the physical pain, there was a feeling. With gallbladders, the feeling is almost always about shame, resentment, and bitterness. I have seen gallbladder problems in women in their forties and fifties who have spent their lives taking care of other people and putting themselves on the back burner. This leads to the feelings of unworthiness and resentment. Before that feeling, perhaps there was a thought, such as *I'm not worthy. I don't deserve to do anything for myself until I take care of everyone else's needs first. I'm not worth the time to take care of myself.*

The resulting feeling, unless released, stays blocked in that organ. The stuck energy of this feeling keeps life-force energy from flowing through the third chakra, and with that comes a lack of blood flow and oxygenation. After a while, you have an organ that doesn't work very well.

As a Reiki practitioner, it's important to begin to learn the emotional and spiritual significance of each part of the body and all the organs. You can read the whole body in this way: the liver holds rage; the kidneys hold fear; and the heart holds grief. There's much to learn by listening to the body. I recommend two books to help with this: *You Can Heal Your Life*, by Louise Hay (1984), and *Your Body Speaks Your Mind*, by Deb Shapiro (2006). These books are fabulous references when learning about how the body holds stuck emotion and energy.

This layering of physical, emotional, and mental issues is where the Reiki Level 2 symbols come in. They have the power to address the levels. If you're working on Susie, who has come to you complaining of her gallbladder issues, you might start by using *Chokurei*, the symbol to release energy on a physical level, on the third chakra, which is the one associated with all digestive issues, including the gallbladder. Then, you might add *Seiheki*, the symbol for emotional healing, to help release stuck emotions. At this point, Susie may get a little angry and begin to cry, both of which are great emotional releases. You might then add *Honshazeshonen*, the symbol to release stuck negative thought patterns. Suddenly, Susie may begin to think that taking care of herself is a good idea after all. This is how powerful Reiki Level 2 can be!

Now that you know where the symbols came from and how they can be used in healing, let's learn about each of them.

Symbol 1: *Chokurei* (CHO-KOO-RAY), Increase Power

Chokurei is the symbol for healing on the physical level. It's meaning is "increase power."

Use it on any physical condition, including that related to pain or trauma. It will bring added energy, or chi, to the spot being worked on, as well as increased blood flow. You can use it for the entire energy system by putting it in the crown of the head, or on any part someone is having trouble with.

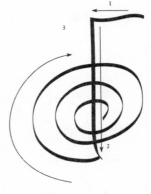

- You can use *Chokurei* on yourself if you're tired. Put it on your forehead for mental clarity and to wake yourself up. You can also do this for others, too.

- Use it on the palms of your hands before you do Reiki to increase the flow of Reiki to your hands.

- Put it on the soles of your feet to help ground yourself. You can do the same thing to your recipient.

- Draw it into the crown to increase energy in general. This is great for people with fatigue issues.

There are some contraindications for *Chokurei*. A contraindication is a time when we don't want to use the symbol because it would not be helpful. Don't use *Chokurei* on a broken bone that hasn't been set yet, since it will begin healing the bone right away, and you don't want the healing to happen until the bone is in the right place. It's fine to use on a bone that has already been set. If you are dealing with someone with a bone break, use plain Reiki without the symbols, or use the symbol *Seiheki* for emotional healing to help calm the person down, at least until the bone has been set.

Chokurei is also contraindicated where there is a known cancer tumor. Since this symbol adds a jolt of energy, we don't want to increase energy to cancer cells in a tumor, which are already growing out of control. Don't dwell too much on the idea that someone might have a tumor that you don't know about, since, in truth, we have things like this in our body all the time that just come and go on their own.

We can use the reverse, or mirror image, of *Chokurei* to take energy out of things. This is good for things like:

- Fever

- A known cancer tumor

- An overbusy mind or insomnia, or both

Don't be afraid to use this symbol even though there are some contraindications. If you stay clear of these few instances, then you will be fine using this very versatile symbol.

Symbol 2: *Seiheki* (SAY-HEY-KEY), Emotional Healing

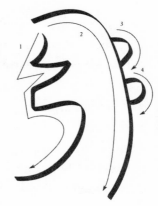

Seiheki is used for emotional healing. Bronwen and Frans Stiene describe the meaning of this symbol as "harmony" (2008), while William Lee Rand describes it as "God and humanity become one" (1998).

Since many illnesses and conditions have an emotional root, this is the symbol you will use frequently. This symbol is great for calming emotional upset. *Seiheki* on the heart, especially the back of the heart, is very good if someone is crying. It will help release the emotional causes of any sickness or condition. *Seiheki* has a sweet and nurturing feeling to it. It's very comforting.

One of the most powerful uses of *Seiheki* is the heart sandwich. This is when we stand at someone's shoulders and put one hand on the front and one on the back of the heart. Flow energy back and forth between your hands after you apply the symbol, and you will feel the person begin to come into balance emotionally. This is one of the best ways to calm an emotional upset, and it may be the most frequently used application of Reiki!

Seiheki is very good at helping you increase your intuition. It can help open people up psychically. Use it on your brow chakra to increase your psychic ability. This symbol activates the pineal gland, which is the seat of psychic insight in your brain. This is why learning Reiki Level 2 and using these symbols increases people's psychic ability so much.

Seiheki is also useful as a sign of protection. Put it on your car or your house as a shield. It protects against negative psychic energy. Some people write it on paper in calligraphy and frame it. If you hang it in a room, it will send healing and protective energy all through your living environment since it's great for clearing out negative energy. There are no contraindications for *Seiheki*, so you can feel very comfortable using it at any time.

Symbol 3: *Honshazeshonen* (HON-SHA-ZAY-SHOW-NEN), Sending Energy Across Distances

This symbol means "sending energy across distances" and can also mean "connection," according to Bronwen and Frans Stiene (2008). It has two main uses. The first way that we use this symbol is for clearing thoughts or mental patterns. It helps release negative thinking or stuck mental concepts. This is a very important step, since our thoughts are part of the equation in the creation of illness and disease.

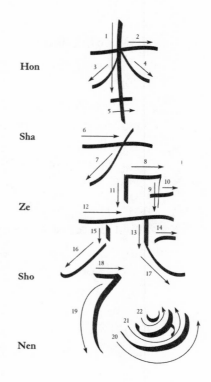

The second way we use this symbol is to send long-distance healing energy. Draw *Honshazeshonen* before you administer the long-distance healing, and then again at the end of the sequence, sandwiching all the other symbols you use between *Honshazeshonen*. *Honshazeshonen* becomes like a set of bookends, with the treatment in between. You'll learn more about long-distance healing later in this chapter.

Learning and Using the Symbols

Before you use the symbols, you need to memorize them—both their names and how to draw them. You can trace them over and over with your finger, saying the name as you do so, or you can use tracing paper. Don't start using them in healing sessions until you are very comfortable saying the name of the symbol (in your head) and drawing it with your finger.

Once you memorize and learn the symbols, here is how you would use the symbols in a healing session:

1. Say the name of the symbol in your head.

2. Draw the symbol on or over the recipient's body in their energy field.

3. Tap the symbol into the energy field three times. Tap right on the place where you placed the symbol. I tap with the finger that I am drawing the symbol with.

Most people use either their index or their middle finger for tapping. You can tap directly on the body, just be gentle. The tap pushes the symbol into the body where it continues to work until the recipients don't need it anymore. The symbol will stay inside their energy field on that spot until they don't need it anymore, and then it just dissolves away. I favor drawing and setting the symbol slightly above the person's skin so you don't tickle them.

How do you know when to use the symbols? With practice, it will become obvious, but even in the beginning common sense will tell you when to use which symbol. Check in with your recipients before you start. If they have physical pain, use *Chokurei*, and if there's an emotional upset, then you'll need *Seiheki*. If you're clear that their thoughts are in the way, then use *Honshazeshonen*.

Your intuition will also help you know when to use the symbols. You may get a sudden impression, urge, or hunch to use a certain symbol. Sometimes the right symbol will just pop into your mind. If so, use it. Your Reiki guides (who we'll learn about a little later) will inspire you to use certain symbols as well. Basically, if a symbol enters your consciousness while you're working on someone, that's your sign to use it.

Practice using the symbols a lot, and you will get to know them. Just as you did while you were learning and practicing Reiki Level 1, use your journal to capture your experiences using the symbols. They each have their own personality, frequency, and energy, and using them frequently and reflecting on them will help you get to know them more deeply and use them more skillfully.

Using the symbols is one way that we get a wonderful opportunity to both notice and increase our psychic impressions. As I noted previously, Reiki Level 2 offers one a substantial increase in intuitive and psychic abilities. I think much of this has to do with the power of the symbol *Seiheki*, which is very effective at opening your psychic gifts.

Your psychic information might take the form of knowing what symbol to use and when to use it. Remember to tune in to your open channel to receive this information. Visual psychics might see an image of the symbol, whereas auditory psychics might hear the name of the symbol in their head. You might have a knowing, a hunch, or a feeling. It's important not to get too hung up on how it's coming and to pay attention.

I have met many talented healers who tell me that they aren't psychic since they never *see* anything. Meanwhile they are receiving tons of valuable information about their recipients on their open channels. If they dismiss this and don't pay attention, then everyone misses out.

Reiki Level 2 Healing Practices

Once you receive the Reiki Level 2 attunement and are comfortable with the three symbols, you are ready to start using them in more formal healing sessions. In this part of the chapter, I'll teach you a variety of things you need to know to work at the Practitioner's Level:

- Hand positions for giving Reiki on a table

- Setting up a dedicated space for giving Reiki

- Conducting the session, including managing client intake and session length

- Managing the emotional energy that comes up for both you and your client

You may still want to offer Reiki more informally, but with the addition of the symbols and with the option of working on a recipient who is lying down on a bed, a table, or the floor. Or, you may work as a nurse, aesthetician, or therapist, or in some other healing vocation, and you will want to find ways to give Reiki in the place or places where you already do your work. Or, you may want to set up a more formal Reiki practice—hanging out your shingle, finding a space and buying a table, and charging for your sessions. Whatever your plans for your Reiki Level 2 skills, you'll find useful principles here.

We'll start with hand positions for a person who is lying on a table and a couple of sequences to use them in. Read this section to learn the sequences, and reread it often for reference as you do more sessions.

ADDING REIKI TO OTHER MODALITIES

Marcia is an aesthetician who has a wonderfully nurturing personality. When I met her, she already had a full practice, and her clients felt loved and restored in her sessions. When she added Reiki Level 2 to her skill set, she began to pause frequently in skin treatments and let the Reiki energy flow through her hands to her clients.

"My hands get so hot, it's like a heating pad for my clients," she said. "They get so much more relaxed, and very quickly too. I now start all my sessions with five minutes of simply holding their heads in my hands until I feel them relax and stop thinking. After that they get so relaxed that they snore and drool on the table. Which is so good for them! It made a big difference in my practice, which doubled after I added Reiki to treatments."

Reiki Level 2 Starter Sequence: Hand Positions for the Table

There are many variations of hand positions in Reiki. In general, we work *down* the body, but, other than that, there's no single right way to work. It's very appropriate to use your intuition to guide your

hand placements. Some schools of Reiki have strict hand placements, but I believe in allowing practitioners to be very flexible and
encourage them to follow their intuition. This approach is particularly beneficial for practitioners who are also developing their psychic,
empathic, and intuitive gifts.

I'm going to teach you some sequences that you can use with
your recipient lying down. As you get familiar with these, it will
become easier for you to branch out and do your own thing when
you feel guided to do so. Remember to be mindful and to take good
notes as you're learning, especially when you try something new, or
work with someone you haven't worked with before.

As always, start with a quick grounding. Do the Reiki breath to
ground and center yourself before you start any Reiki session, and set
your intention to turn Reiki on. Your recipient should be lying on his
or her back, with limbs relaxed.

It's nice to offer a pillow or bolster under the knees to support the
lower back and a small pillow under the heads, since most people
find it uncomfortable to lie completely flat on their back. Offer a
blanket, too, since we tend to lower our body temperature as we
relax, and people can get cold during a session. Eye pillows are useful
for people with busy minds, since closing our eyes tends to relax the
mind. I use one that has some lavender flowers mixed in, and I sandwich it in a tissue, which I dispose of at the end of the session.

As you learned in Reiki Level 1, bridge positions connect one
chakra to another, so one hand is on one chakra and the other hand
is on another one, creating a connection, or bridge, between the two
chakras. This brings balance to the chakras and creates energy flow
throughout the system. I find this sequence to be especially good for
someone who is feeling anxious and disconnected.

Hold each position until you feel the energy crescendo, which we
discussed in chapter 5. Be flexible with how long this takes. Some
people spend about five minutes on each position, but I prefer to feel
what is happening in the moment with the client. In some positions,
you will feel the energetic release right away, and then it's okay to
move your hands. Other places will feel more stuck, and you might
need to keep your hands in one place for ten minutes to feel the
energy crescendo and corresponding energy release.

This is a great time to let your intuition and your inner guidance direct you. Chances are very good that you will perceive when to move your hands based on this guidance. I feel so much in my own body, so I am constantly paying attention to what is happening with my breath and my own energy system.

HANDSHAKE POSITION

Begin with the handshake position. (This is when your hands are on the recipient's shoulders.) You can either sit or stand at the head of the table. Use your guidance to tell you how long to stay there and wait for the feeling of connecting with your client.

FIRST HEAD POSITION

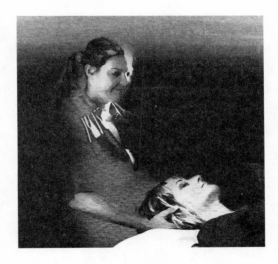

Place both hands under the back of the head. Wait here until you feel your client's thinking slow down. This might be the most important position you can do! Clients will relax a lot once they can stop the overthinking. Look for a corresponding exhale in your client.

CROWN AND BROW BRIDGE POSITION

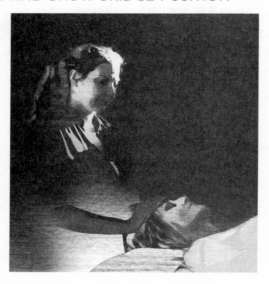

Place both palms on the crown, fingers on the brow. Do your best to connect these two chakras with the intention to flow energy back and forth between them to balance them. This position also calms the mind.

TEMPLE SANDWICH

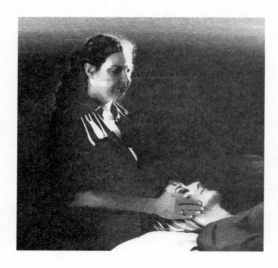

Place your palms on the temples, with the fingertips facing down the jawline. Move the energy back and forth between your hands. This balances the energy flowing through the brain and begins to balance the hemispheres of the brain. For a variation, place the palm over the brow, fingers over the face, avoiding the nose and mouth. This is a great position for people who have trouble with their eyes or sinus issues since the Reiki energy is directed to the eyes and sinuses in this position.

THROAT AND HEART BRIDGE

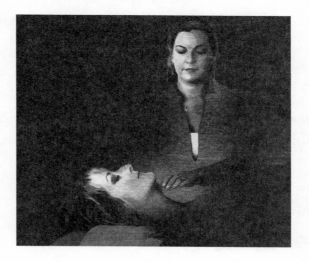

Stand or sit at the client's shoulder with one hand under the back of the neck and one hand hovering over the top of the neck. Don't touch the front of the neck, or your client will feel like you are throttling him or her. This chakra is balanced when you feel the energy flowing evenly between your hands.

Now, bridge the throat and heart. Keep your *top* hand (the one closest to your client's head) on the back of the neck, and your *bottom* hand (the hand nearest the client's feet) on the heart. Watch your hand placement on the heart, working high up on the breastbone if you're working on a woman. If you're working on a man, the heart chakra is right at the center of the chest.

HEART AND SOLAR PLEXUS BRIDGE

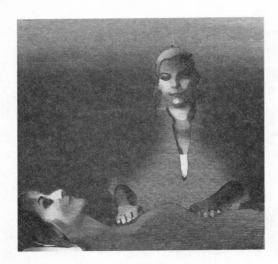

Place one hand on the heart and one hand at the solar plexus, bridging the two. Run the Reiki energy back and forth between your hands until you feel the energy run smoothly. This position calms anxiety.

SOLAR PLEXUS AND NAVEL BRIDGE

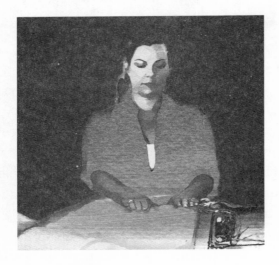

Place one hand on the second chakra and one hand on the third chakra, connecting them. Watch your hand position on the navel. Work on the belt line for a woman and above the belt line for a man. Never touch anyone near or below the pubic bone.

It's nice to throw in a sandwich position here, too. To do this on the navel, for example, put one hand under the body with your palm flat on the sacrum, and the top hand goes palm down on the lower belly. You can easily get your hand under the body by lifting the edge of the sheet to roll the person slightly onto one hip, just enough to get your hand under the client. Press your hand down into the padding of the table and slide your hand between the person and the table. It's best to take your rings and bracelets off for this!

NAVEL AND ROOT BRIDGE

You can easily access the first chakra at the knees, so place your top hand on the second chakra at the navel, and move your bottom hand so that it is resting on one or both knees. Feel free to spend a lot of time here, since it is a very grounding position and most people need help and extra time to feel grounded. You can aid this by really concentrating on being grounded yourself. Connect to the grounding cord and breathe. As you ground yourself, you will remind your client what it feels like to be more grounded, too.

ARMS

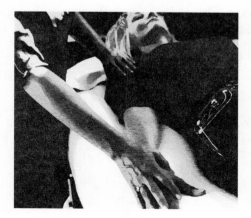

Working down the arms, do each arm individually with the top hand on the shoulder and the bottom hand on the client's hand, as if you are holding hands. We often store grief in the arms, since they are connected to the heart chakra. You can also do each part of the arm separately—just the shoulders, just the elbow, or just the hand. Don't forget to do both sides!

LEGS

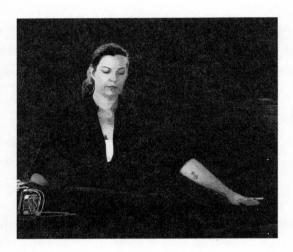

Working down the legs, place your top hand on the outer hip and your bottom hand as far down the leg as you can reach. Think about flowing energy down the leg and giving the person a chance to ground. Sometimes the legs feel very cold or stiff, almost as if they are made of wood. This is a sign that the person is not very grounded and may have an energetic habit of being "out" of the legs. Work both legs until they feel warm and the energy is flowing easily down both legs. Touch only the outer edge of the legs. Never touch the inside of someone's legs, especially from the knee up to the groin.

FEET: FINISH AND GROUND

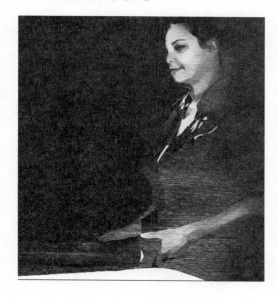

Finish the session by holding the feet. Stand at the foot of the table and hold on to the instep of each foot. Ground yourself while you're doing this. It's good to have a slight flexion in your knees and to breathe deeply and slowly and to encourage the client to ground as deeply as possible. Step slowly away from the client to break the connection. You can allow clients to stay on the table for a few minutes to help them integrate the session, rather than rushing them off the table. It's a good idea to remind them to sit up slowly since many people become light-headed if they jump off the table too quickly.

It's normal to feel a little spacey and relaxed after a Reiki session. I call this "Reiki head," and you want to make sure clients are grounded enough to drive home safely before they leave your office. Let them talk about their experience a little bit, and give them a glass of water to drink.

Don't forget to ground and clear yourself when the session is over. Drop anything that you picked up during the session by dropping it down the grounding cord with your breath.

This bridge sequence is wonderful for bringing balance to the person receiving it. The next sequence is a series of sandwich positions to work the front and back aspect of the chakras at the same time.

Working Down the Back

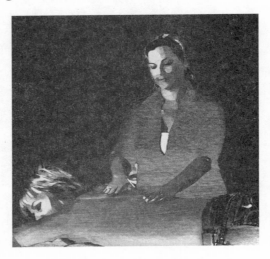

After completing the front sequence, you can also work on the back of a person. Have the client turn over. (You need a face cradle on the table to do this properly. Line the face cradle with tissues, paper towels, or a face cradle cover that you can wash afterward.) Start with your hands on the shoulders in the handshake position:

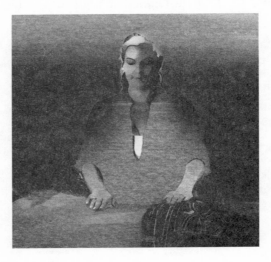

1. Hover over the back of the head to get the back of the brow chakra. You can also work the back of the neck very easily here, too.

2. Work on the back of the heart.

3. Work on the back of the solar plexus.

4. Move to the sacrum.

5. Then, move down the back of the legs.

6. Hold the feet, and you're done.

Reiki Level 2 Sandwich Position Sequence for the Table

This sequence works both sides of the body at once. It's very thorough and efficient. It's a great choice if you want a thorough healing and you only have a little time. As always, connect with the grounding cord to ground and center yourself before you start working, and turn Reiki on. You can place your hands on the shoulders for the handshake position before you start this sequence.

HEAD

1. Start with your hands under the back of the client's head to slow down the person's thinking.

2. Move to the side of the table and leave one hand under the back of the head and the other hand over the brow in the sixth-chakra sandwich. Sitting in a chair is helpful. If you are standing, make sure your posture is as upright as you can get it. Leaning over the table can hurt your back, so you need to practice good body mechanics when you are doing Reiki.

THROAT CHAKRA

1. Sitting or standing at the client's shoulder, put one hand on the back of the neck with the other hand hovering over the throat.

2. Never touch the front of the throat.

HEART CHAKRA

1. Sandwich the front and back of the heart by placing one hand underneath the client between the shoulder blades, and the top hand on the breastbone, if you are working on a woman, or at the center of the chest, if you are working on a man. Watch your hand placement when working on the chest of a woman.

2. Move the energy back and forth between your hands until you feel the front and back of the chakras balance.

SOLAR PLEXUS CHAKRA

1. The lower hand goes to the back of the solar plexus, where the bra strap would be. The top hand rests lightly on the solar plexus. Most people are very blocked in this chakra, as it's the chakra of self-esteem and self-worth. If the client has poor self-esteem, it will feel very blocked.

2. When the energy releases you should feel a change in respiration. Breathing will slow down and deepen when this chakra clears since your hands are often sending energy right through the diaphragm. Ask your client to breathe deeply from the diaphragm to release stuck energy.

NAVEL CHAKRA

1. Place one hand under the body with the palm holding the sacrum. The top hand goes on the lower belly. You can hover over the lower belly or touch at about the belt buckle. Be

sensitive to where your hands are, and remember to work with your eyes open.

2.   This chakra holds blocked emotions, and it can take time for it to release.

FEET AND FINISH

1.   To finish, stand at the foot of the table and hold on to both feet. Ground yourself by connecting to the grounding cord. This helps your client remember what being grounded feels like.

2.   Once you feel complete here, step away from the table and take a moment to recenter yourself. Put your hands on your heart to come back to yourself. Do the Reiki breath again or try the Reiki Waterfall Exercise to help you let go of anything that you might have picked up in the session.

3.   Let the client rest on the table for a few minutes and help them to get up slowly.

Reiki Level 2 Spread-and-Bridge Sequence for the Table

Another good pattern is to alternate spreads and bridges. This works wonders if someone is experiencing poor health, since the spread positions work inside the muscle and organ tissues of the body, while the bridge positions work the chakras. Remember, a spread position is done with your hands across the body, rather than on the midline of the body where the chakra is.

1.   To begin, work whichever head positions seem appropriate. When you get to the heart, do the heart spread with your hands spread across the chest. This will send energy to the heart and lungs.

2.   Next, do the heart and solar plexus bridge to connect those chakras.

3. Follow that with the solar plexus spread. This sends Reiki to the organs of the digestive area, such as the liver, gallbladder, stomach, pancreas, and spleen. This is wonderful for digestive complaints.

4. Now do the solar plexus and navel bridge.

5. Then, do the navel spread, covering the lower digestive and reproductive organs.

6. Next, do the navel and root bridge.

7. Close by holding the feet to ground the client.

You now have some useful sequences to start practicing Reiki on people who are lying on a table. As you gain more and more experience doing Reiki this way, you will find that you naturally vary these sequences as your intuition guides you.

Your Healing Space

Whether you are working on a table or in a chair, it's important to create a quiet, healing space to do your Reiki sessions in. Depending on the context where you do your work, you might or might not be able to have a dedicated space to do Reiki. Wherever you work, it's important to energetically prepare the room before doing energy work.

• Smudge with sage or burn incense.

• Let in some light and fresh air.

• Say a prayer or set an intention.

Smudging with sage clears the room of leftover energy, so you can start with clear energy. A prayer or intention setting will also help you to create a sacred space in your healing room. You can do whatever kind of prayer or intention resonates for you, anything from the Lord's Prayer to a personal mantra.

If you can set up a dedicated space as a Reiki treatment room, it should be quiet and peaceful. Here is the essential equipment for a dedicated Reiki room:

- Massage table

- Two comfortable chairs, plus an extra folding chair

- Tissue boxes

- Clock or timer of some kind (I have three in my small office so I can see the time no matter where I'm standing, and my client can, too.)

- Sage and a lighter, or a spray, for clearing the space between client sessions

- Eye pillows, a bolster, and a variety of other pillows for people who need props on the table

- A variety of blankets and sheets to help regulate the temperature of clients

- A sturdy step stool for people who need assistance getting onto the table

- File cabinet for client notes and intake forms

- Clipboard and pens for intake forms

- Music or a sound machine

Anything else is up to you; have fun personalizing your space! Notice that many of these suggested items can move with you if your Reiki healing takes you outside of your dedicated space.

Getting a Reiki Table

By the time you've reached Reiki Level 2, you've probably graduated from chair Reiki and want to move on to something more like a proper Reiki session, with your clients lying on a massage table in a room dedicated to your Reiki practice.

It's very bad for your back to try and do Reiki with someone lying on the floor or on a regular bed, although in a pinch you can do it anywhere if you really need to. There are many massage tables out there, so you have many options to choose from. You can get very fancy, expensive ones, or you can get one at Sam's Club or Costco, which sometimes have great deals. Many people buy them online at places like Massage Warehouse, or even Amazon.

Getting one used is a great idea if you're trying to save money, so check out places like Craigslist for used items. You can often find a whole setup there for under $100.

Here are some things to think about if you're going to invest in a table:

- Weight is very important if you're going to be moving it around. Try to get one that is thirty-five pounds or less.

- You need a carrying case if you're going to transport it. You may want to take it to a client's house or a Reiki share.

- You need a head cradle, too. Consider a package that has the table, the head cradle, the carrying case, and, sometimes, a bolster for one price.

- It should be rated to hold at least five hundred pounds. (More is even better; I saw one collapse with three people sitting on it during a Reiki class.)

- You can get special sheets for it, but twin sheets work just fine.

- Tables with metal legs are often lighter than tables with wooden ones.

- You can get a heavy, solid table if you know you're never going to move it, but most people do end up moving theirs at some point.

Doing an Intake

Doing an intake just means that you are checking in with your clients before your session, which is always important to do. The intake lets you know what's happening with them in general, and at that moment.

I usually start with the simple questions "How are you feeling today? What's bringing you in for a session?" You want to find out how they're feeling and what they want in their session. They almost always know and are happy to tell you. Here are some things I've heard clients say:

- I'm totally stressed. I just need to relax.

- I have a horrible headache today.

- I just ended a relationship and I need help letting it go.

- I just want to try Reiki. I've heard so much about it!

- I'm here because you said you needed to practice!

Aside from getting a sense of why they're there and what they need and want from the session, it's a good idea to ask some additional follow-up questions to guide your session. You need to know these things:

- Is there a crisis of some kind?

- Do you have any major medical issues?

- Is there an emotional issue that is upsetting you?

- Do you have any mental health issues? Are you on any psychiatric medications?

- Do you know what you need and want in the session today?

If you are going to have a formal Reiki practice with paying clients, it is essential to have intake and consent forms that your clients sign before each session. I recommend that you take notes after the session to record what happened the session. All professional body workers are trained to do this so we can keep accurate records of our ongoing work with our clients. Please see http://www .newharbinger.com/41214 for downloadable copies of these forms.

Practice Consensual and Safe Touch

During a Reiki session, always ask permission before touching a client. This includes casual hugs and pats. Simply ask, "Are you comfortable being touched?" or "Can I give you a hug?" and then act accordingly. Every person has the right to refuse touch and to expect only permission-based touch. Never override clients' wishes, make assumptions, or make them feel weird about it. This is especially true if you're working with a child. Remember, you can do an entire Reiki session working with your hands off the body. If you are granted permission to touch your client's body, obviously there are places we can touch and places that we can't: Do not touch anyone's breasts or genitals. Ever. Here are some guidelines to follow for consensual and safe touch:

- You can touch the outside of the leg all the way from the outer hip down to the feet. You can touch the inner leg from the ankle to the knee.

- Do not touch the inside of the leg from knee to groin.

- Do not touch below the belt line on men. When you are working on a man, you work the second chakra at the belt, never below it.

- Do not touch the pubic bone on women, or go any lower than that.

- Do not offer sexual touching, come-ons, or innuendos, ever.

- Never date your clients. It's essential to have good boundaries around our sexuality when we are healers.

I have witnessed a lot of touch violations by well-meaning practitioners who were working with their eyes completely shut, and then trying to move around the client's body by feeling around. Please don't do this. Put yourself in the client's shoes and imagine how you would feel if that was happening to you.

Considerations for Scheduling and Running a Session

There are a lot of variations for the length and rhythm of a session, and you can do your sessions any way that you want to. If you are doing a formal Reiki healing session as a Reiki practitioner, I recommend scheduling hour-long appointments, or, at the most, an hour and a half. Keeping to your time is a very important part of keeping healthy boundaries, so don't go more than a few minutes over it if you can avoid it.

If you plan an hour-long session, ten to fifteen minutes will be used for intake and thirty to forty minutes for Reiki healing. When you are finished, make sure to also do a very quick check-in with your clients. It's better not to talk directly to them too much after the healing. You can follow up during the intake at their next session. If you talk a lot at the end of the appointment, you'll bring them out of their state of healing and put them back into their heads. Thinking too much will diminish the results of the Reiki.

You spend a lot of time getting your clients out of their thinking mind so they can let the energy flow. They'll go into an altered state during the session as their brain waves shift from beta state (busy mind) to the alpha and theta states (healing). This is what we mean when we say a client is *in state*. The longer we can keep them there after the healing, the better.

I know practitioners who leave their clients on the table for five to ten minutes after a healing, with music playing and an eye pillow on. They go outside the room, write up their notes, and then come back in. I think this is a lovely way to end a session.

Find a gentle way to let your clients know the session is over. I sometimes use sage, and either spray or burn it (make sure your clients don't have sensitivities). Some practitioners use a chime or bell, or they simply turn the music down or off. You can also put your hand on their shoulder and bring them back gently by saying something like "Okay, our session is over. Please take a minute and then get up slowly."

It's very important to have your clients get off the table very slowly. People are often light-headed after a Reiki treatment. Have them sit on the edge of the table until they are sure of their balance. You don't want to have someone fall in your office, and there's no reason this should happen if you prepare your clients properly. This is what I say to my clients: "Please, sit up very slowly. You might be light-headed, which is totally normal after a Reiki treatment. Don't jump off the table until you find your feet."

You'll find your own style and rhythm to doing a healing session, and that's a beautiful thing.

Handling an Emotional Release

If you are doing Reiki sessions, it's only a matter of time before a recipient has a big emotional release during a session. This is good! It's a huge benefit to the client and one of the most healing things that can happen in a session.

An emotional release can look like a lot of things. The client might cry, laugh, want to talk through something, or even shake. It can be quite dramatic, like emotional hysterics, or it can very subtle, like twitching, breathing changes, or trembling. It's very important to feel comfortable with your client's emotional release, so you can encourage it. If you are not comfortable with it as a practitioner, your client will unconsciously feel that and hold back an emotional release.

If you are trained as a counselor, you will know what to do. But many Reiki practitioners don't have formal psychological training, and yet we still need to know how to help our clients through an intense emotional release when it happens.

Most of my clients cry on my table. I think we all hold in our feelings way too much, and Reiki gets that energy flowing. I think it's very healthy and much needed to release in this way. That's why I give tacit energetic permission to my clients to let it rip!

Here are some guidelines to help you skillfully navigate a client through an emotional release.

Let the Client Lead

Unless you are a trained counselor, let the client lead the way. We all have inner wisdom that governs our healing process, and clients usually know what they need and what's beneficial and comfortable for them. I let my clients lead the way into deep emotional water, but only if it comes up for them. If my clients start crying, I will ask them to breathe deeply and allow the energy to move through their body.

I will ask, "What's coming up for you?" Then, I listen without attachment to what is emerging for them.

They might say something like "I feel so sad about my divorce! I thought I was over it. I am so angry, and I don't know why."

If you stay curious and nonjudgmental, they will usually be able to work their own way through it. Often, I say nothing and let them process it in their own time. Or, I will ask gentle, open-ended questions, such as:

- Where does that feeling come from?

- What do you need to do to let that go?

- What do you need right now?

What we don't want to do is lead them into deep emotional water on our own and uncover things that they are not ready to handle in the moment. Don't poke around the deep past of their childhood or stir up unresolved trauma unless they bring it up first. Leave that to the trained counselors and therapists.

This is where empaths shine, so don't forget to tune in to your client's feelings during a session. This is what being an empath is for, so this is the perfect time to use your empathic gifts. Tune in to yourself too, since what you are feeling is likely a clue to what your client might be feeling.

In one of my sessions, a client was telling me how horrible her divorce was. She was holding herself very stiffly, trying to speak logically about it, and I had this sudden and strong urge to stand up, scream, and throw my teacup across the room. This intense feeling came out of nowhere, but I knew it was her feeling since I don't usually feel that way when I am working. I said, "You seem very calm about it. I think I would be very angry. Are you angry?" It was good to see the mask crack, and she was finally able to let out her anger in a healthy way.

Constantly monitoring your own emotions and physical sensations during your time with your Reiki recipients will give you a lot of potentially useful information about what is going on with them. It's also important to be mindful about our boundaries so that we are not picking up and holding on to the recipient's physical or emotional pain. You only need to experience it for a few seconds, long enough to identify it, and then you can flush it down the grounding cord using your breath. No need to bring it home with you.

Get Them to Breathe

We are all used to holding our breath when we are trying to shut down a powerful feeling. It's a habit most of us learn in childhood to avoid crying in public. I carefully watch to make sure my clients are not holding their breath or breathing in a very shallow way.

When big emotions come up, they move through us like waves. If we allow clients to fully let that wave move all the way through them, the emotion will resolve easily on its own. When we hold back the wave, the feeling sticks around for a long time and creates problems and blocks in the energy field, chakras, and the body. Plus, it feels terrible.

When I sense a strong emotion coming up, I ask clients to breathe deeply into the emotion, directing their breath to the part of the body that is holding the emotion. Then, I recommend that they breathe the feeling out of their body in any way that feels natural to them. The exhale breath allows the energy of the emotion to leave the body, which is the desired outcome here.

Some people want to breathe up from their toes and exhale out their mouth. Other people will breathe in through their mouth and release the emotional energy down their legs and out the bottom of their feet. I suggest both ways and let clients choose. If the breath is used to release the emotional energy, most people can clear even a very strong feeling in a few minutes. These waves of emotion don't last longer than a few minutes if we really allow the energy to move through us.

Use Active and Reflective Listening Skills

Powerful healing happens when we show up as a compassionate witness to someone else's pain. When we stay present with people as they go through their process, we give them a great gift—the gift of not being alone in their pain as they shine a light into their dark places. Many people want to talk about their emotional release, so be prepared for this. It's so beneficial and healing for someone to express their emotions and just be heard. Do your best to encourage this. Again, unless you are a trained counselor, you are going to stick with active and reflective listening skills. This allows the clients to unfold their experience at their own pace. We support them, but we don't interfere or lead them deeper than they are ready to go.

Active listening sounds just like what it is. It means really listening to what someone is saying. Validation is a huge part of active listening. Most people just want to have their feelings heard and acknowledged. They want to be told that their feelings are normal. Being deeply listened to and validated is an incredibly healing experience for most people.

Here are some examples of what you might say to someone expressing feelings:

I hear what you're saying. That must have been really hard.

Of course you feel angry. Anyone would in that situation.

I can really hear how sad you are right now. It's okay if you want to cry. I don't mind.

Reflective listening is reflecting back to clients what they're saying and how they're feeling. Sometimes they don't know that they're having a feeling. We are so conditioned to shut them down that we don't even know we're having them. Reflective listening is good for helping people tune in to and integrate their feelings.

Here are a few more examples of how to respond:

Sounds like you're pretty confused and angry right now.

So, what I hear you saying is that you're really scared of not knowing what's coming next.

Everyone feels afraid when they face the unknown. That's not unusual at all.

Adding Your Insight

Adding an insight or two is good in small measure. Your intuitive and empathic gifts will give you lots of information during a session, and sometimes you get a hint of something your clients are going through, but they don't know it yet themselves. This is where it pays to be very careful. For instance, you may get a hit that their pain is related to past abuse, but they haven't linked the two yet. You'll have to tread carefully here. Or, you just "know" that a divorce is in their immediate future because you can see it coming from a mile away, but if they're not ready to hear that yet, you can cause more harm than good by telling them before they're ready for it.

The best insight to share is the one that they're just about to figure out for themselves anyway. Insight is best when it comes naturally to you, and it would be what you would say to anyone in that situation. Insight is often something common sense that they just can't see right now. Think about the advice that you would give your best friend in the same situation.

You might say something like "It sounds like you really need to take care of yourself right now. This is a big piece of work you are doing right now. I feel like you need more support than you are getting now. Have you thought about seeing a therapist?"

When we put active and reflective listening together with our insight, we can really help our clients. It's like a recipe:

- Sixty percent active listening

- Thirty percent reflecting back to them

- Ten percent adding your own two cents

Sharing Your Psychic Hits

The more we practice Reiki, especially when we mix it with psychic development, the more hits we get. This is a good thing! But, with this power comes responsibility. As you get used to picking up psychic information during your sessions, it's important to learn how to best add this into your conversations with your clients.

You may be seeing things, feeling things, or "just knowing" things. You might be seeing colors around your clients. Or you might be getting a straight-up vision of Mother Mary giving you the low-down on your client. It can be nerve-racking to try to get enough confidence to share your hits with your clients, but if you ask permission before you share a hit, and offer the information you received *without interpreting it for your client*, you will be able to use your hits safely and effectively.

As psychics with good ethics, we always ask for permission to share our hits, both inside and outside of sessions. It's very bad form to spring psychic information on someone who hasn't asked for it, despite what you see TV psychics do. It's a horrible boundary violation, *especially* when you're not in a session. So, we *always* ask. You might say, "I got a hit while I was working on you. Do you want me to share it with you?" This is all you need say, and chances are good that they'll say yes. If they don't, then please keep it to yourself.

If you perceive something, try to share it without your interpretation. Newbie psychics make the mistake of trying to tell people what they personally think the meaning of their insight is. You'll be much more helpful if you don't. You never know what things mean to other people.

When I was very young, I got a strange vision in a session. I was doing readings at a psychic fair and would have my clients sit in a chair. I would then stand behind them and put my hands on their shoulders, since I get a stronger reading on someone when I'm touching them. When I touched one woman, I immediately saw a bowl of tangerines on a wooden table. I could smell the tangerines and see the details of their color, and then I felt a huge wave of sadness wash over me.

I thought, *A bowl of tangerines? You have got to be kidding me.* I could not find any meaning to this vision myself. I explained what I had seen and felt without adding my own interpretation, simply because I couldn't find one. I asked my client if it meant anything to her. She burst into tears and told me that she was looking for a sign from her mother who had passed away when she was a child. When her father came in to tell her that her mother had died, there had been a bowl of tangerines on the wooden kitchen table. She said she could never eat tangerines after that because they reminded her so strongly of her mother's death, and that she even hated the smell of them. It was the perfect sign that she was looking for. But, it had meant nothing to me, and there was no way I could have interpreted it without her input.

Know Your Limits and Refer Out

Sometimes we encounter a situation with clients we are not equipped to deal with. Serious mental or physical health issues, trauma, and addictions require that clients also work with people who are experts on these issues. If you uncover something like this in a session, refer them to a specialist. I have a big network of practitioners and specialists whom I refer my clients to when they have something that is beyond my scope. I have business cards for people whose work I know and respect. I network with:

- Chiropractors

- Acupuncturists

- Nutritionists

- Counselors and therapists

- Couples therapists

- Addiction counselors

- Trauma counselors

- Functional medicine doctors

Anyone who has a mental health issue, is taking medication, or has been hospitalized for mental health issues, should also be working in conjunction with their regular therapist. When you do your intake, find out what your client's mental state is and whether he or she has any other medical conditions that would require you to be cautious doing Reiki.

Do Your Own Inner Work

It's vital to continue to do your own inner work. We can only go to those emotional depths with our clients if we are comfortable and willing to go there ourselves. If you're uneasy with your own emotions, then you'll feel uneasy with other people's emotions. If you can't tolerate your own pain, then you won't be able to tolerate other people's pain. If you want to deepen your connection to your client's emotional processes, take the time to do your own inner work.

As healers, our business depends on us continuing to do our own inner-growth work. A healer's business will dry up if he stops doing his inner work. We are always our own first and best clients. Due to the law of resonance, you will attract clients who have your same issues. It's very common for me to see several clients every week who walk in the door with an issue I may also be experiencing. This is one of the things that I like best about being a healer. It keeps me on the edge of my own inner work, so that I am always continuing to grow.

It's important for you to have your own team of healers to work with. Everyone responds to different modalities and healers, so explore until you find what works for you. I recommend someone to talk to, like a therapist or coach, as well as some form of body work.

I go regularly to the massage therapist and I do love acupuncture, too. I highly recommend that you get regular energy work done yourself—get plenty of Reiki! It's fun to find another Reiki practitioner with whom you can trade sessions regularly.

Doing your own inner work is so important; it may be the most important part of your practice. It's truly the difference between the practitioner who has a line of clients begging for sessions and the one who has an empty office. You need to be someone your clients trust and feel confident about working with; someone who has walked a little further down the path than they have. If you are a train wreck in your own life, it's not much of an inspiration for your clients. This doesn't mean you need to be perfect, and have already reached enlightenment, it just means you should always be in the process of healing. It's a continual process.

Long-Distance Healing

Long-distance healing is the ability to send Reiki over distances, and it's a fantastic benefit of learning Reiki Level 2. There's no limit to how much Reiki you can send, and it doesn't matter how far away the recipient is. This is beneficial for friends and relatives who live far away and need some love or healing energy. I also use it like a prayer. When I see an ambulance zoom by or hear a sad story on the news, I send Reiki. It's empowering to know that we can help for people we don't know, even in remote places. You can also use long-distance Reiki with someone who's in the same room with you, but whom you can't touch. Like teachers who can't touch their students or therapists who can't touch their clients.

Ask Permission

We must always ask permission to send long-distance Reiki, just as we do when we are offering it in person. Ask, "Would you like some Reiki? It's a very gentle but powerful energy healing technique from Japan. Can I send you some long distance?"

If they say no, it's very important to respect that. Sending energy against someone's wishes violates personal boundaries. There are times when we want to send Reiki but can't ask the receiver since they aren't available to us in real time. You can't very well stop the ambulance that's zooming by to ask the people inside if they would like to receive Reiki! If people are not available to ask, then ask on the soul level. Simply close your eyes, tune in, and ask if it's in their highest interest to receive the healing energy of Reiki in this moment. You will get some kind of affirmation. Some people hear or see the words yes or no. Others see the person in their mind's eye nod and smile or turn away. Some people just get a strong sense of knowing the right answer.

If you get a strong *no*, don't send Reiki! No means no, even in Reiki. When you get a *yes*, you are free to go ahead and send Reiki. If you receive an inconclusive answer, send Reiki anyway, with this caveat in mind: for the highest good of all and with harm to none. In this case, make sure you send out the intention that if it's not in that person's best interest to receive Reiki, then may it go to whomever needs it most. Or, you can send it directly to the earth to be absorbed.

Check Your Agenda

I have seen people pray and send Reiki to try and *force* someone to get better so that they'll live. Living or dying, healing or not healing, is between that person and the Divine. It's really none of our business, even when it's someone we're close to. As healers, we need to let go of our judgment that living is better than dying.

Dr. Albert Schweitzer, a medical doctor and a philosopher who wrote about the philosophy of healing and medicine, said, "There is a cure for every illness, if you consider death a cure." If you're working with clients at the end of life, chances are good that they will use the Reiki energy to help them cross over and die, not to heal and live. That's a wonderful use of Reiki if that is what needs to happen. It's our own need for the person to live, and our own fear of grief or death that creates an agenda in us that says living is better than dying. Of course, if it's someone close to you, you're not going to want them to die; that's just human nature and perfectly normal. But, it's important to check in with yourself and make sure that you're not holding on to them too much. You need to find a way to process your own feelings about it.

Be mindful of using a lot of Reiki and prayer on someone to stop them from doing something that you don't approve of. You should not use Reiki to take away someone's free will about anything, even if you think it's for their own good. This is a kind of *black magic* dressed up in Reiki to try and *make* someone else be something we want them to be, or to change who they are on the inside. We should never use prayer or Reiki to try and change someone's free will at any level.

I worked with a young man whose very religious parents had a mass said every week to try and stop him from being gay and to "save" his soul. But, it felt like an energy attack to him, and it was. Once, I had to convince a well-meaning mother that it was wrong to send long-distance Reiki to her daughter to keep her from moving across the country, because the mother felt her daughter was making the wrong choice. When you're sending Reiki, check your agenda at the door and ask for it to serve the "highest good of all," with the deep understanding that you probably have no idea what that is.

How to Heal from a Distance

There are several different ways to do long-distance healing. There's no wrong way to do it, so just find one that suits you or feel free to make up your own. One of the great things about long-distance Reiki is that it takes less time than a regular Reiki session. Don't underestimate the power of doing even five minutes of long-distance Reiki for someone!

I list the various methods below, but no matter what method you use, follow these guidelines:

- Check your motivation.

- Get permission, either directly or indirectly.

- If you can, agree on a time.

- Have your Reiki recipients lie down somewhere comfortable. It's very important to agree on a time and to get

them to relax somewhere. You wouldn't want to start working on them while they were driving, or doing anything that required their full attention.

- Start and stop with *Honshazeshonen.*

- Call the recipient after the session and find out how it went. It's fun to share experiences!

Do Reiki on Yourself as You Imagine the Other Person

Sit in a chair and call the person to mind. Start with the symbol *Honshazeshonen.* Draw it in the air and then proceed to do Reiki on yourself while you hold the image of the recipient in your mind. Finish with *Honshazeshonen* to complete your long-distance session. This method has a nice advantage of offering you some Reiki as well.

Use a Proxy

Again, starting with *Honshazeshonen,* use a proxy, such as a doll or a teddy bear, to start the session. Do Reiki on the proxy as if it is the person. Finish with *Honshazeshonen.* When my kids were very young, I used to do this with their teddy bears and then give them the bears to hold. You can also use a doll or anything else that is mostly human in shape.

The Small Hands Technique

Hold out one hand and imagine that the person is so small that she fits in your palm. Start with *Honshazeshonen* and then do Reiki on her whole body, as if she was in your hands. You can use whatever symbols you would like. Finish with *Honshazeshonen.* This gives recipients Reiki all over their body at once.

Sit in a Chair and Imagine the Recipient's Head Is in Your Lap

This is how I work with people who ask for long-distance healing as part of a professional session. I imagine that their head is resting on my knees, and I go through the hand positions without moving but imagining that they're moving under my hands. Always begin and end a long-distance session with *Honshazeshonen*.

Imagine the Client is on Your Reiki Table

If you have a Reiki table set up, you can imagine that your clients are lying on it, and you can go through the positions as if they're really on the table. Imagine that you're touching them. I do this on my Reiki table and run through the hand positions as if there is really someone on my table. Use a bolster and pillows so it feels like there is a real person on the table.

The Takeaway

I hope you feel very comfortable now with Reiki Level 2. At this level, you learned the Reiki Level 2 symbols and how to use them. This gives you the ability to do healing work on a physical, emotional, and mental level with your recipients. Once you learned the symbols and how to use them, we delved into a few of my favorite hand positions for working with someone who is lying on a Reiki table. We also covered how to establish a thoughtful and ethical healing practice that includes how to run a Reiki session and how to set up your healing space so that your Reiki recipients feel safe and welcomed.

Then, you learned how to effectively handle a client's emotional release and to understand when to refer your clients to other practitioners. Knowing this can help us feel skilled and confident when things get deep in a Reiki session, especially because that is what we want to have happen. We wrapped up the chapter with methods and protocols for doing long-distance healing sessions.

Most people have a dramatic increase in their psychic ability when they learn Reiki Level 2. In the next chapter, we'll talk about how to continue to cultivate your psychic abilities and how to get to know and learn to work with your Reiki guides. Working with your guides can be the most fulfilling and exciting part of the Reiki Level 2 training.

CHAPTER 7

Safe Psychic Development and Working with Your Reiki Guides

Most people experience a dramatic increase in both their intuition and their psychic ability at Reiki Level 2. As you are working on your Level 2 skills, it's a good time to learn to take advantage of the information you are getting from your intuitive and psychic gifts. As discussed in the first chapter of this book, being psychic is a natural part of the human experience. It's part of our birthright as human beings.

When we are opening psychically, one of the first things that we need to address is fear. You might be one of the rare few who have no fear attached to being psychic, and, if so, that's great! However, most people are frightened of some aspect of being psychic. Media portrayals of the spiritual or energy realms are often scary, and we have all seen horror movies where things don't go too well for the poor psychics.

Perhaps you had scary psychic experiences in your past, and so you decided to shut down your psychic insight. Psychic children sometimes shut down their abilities because they perceived something that frightened them or someone else. These kids shut down and get scared because and they don't have the language or the support system to help them understand what happened.

The following story is a great example of someone who was very psychic as a child and had to shut down her abilities because they caused great fear in the people around her. Fortunately, she had the courage to step into her gift as an adult, and, in doing so, she healed her past.

❀ *Rosalie's Story* ❀
Psychic, Not Psychotic

Rosalie was from an older generation, and all the people in her family were devout Catholics. She was about sixty years old when she came to my psychic development class, and she had a lot of fear about opening up her abilities.

As a child, she had been very psychic, seeing angels and hearing the voices of her dead relatives. She frequently had dreams that came true. When she was a teen, her psychic experiences increased, which is completely normal for a psychic. But, her mother took her to the doctor out of concern. Rosalie told the doctor everything, about the angels and the voices. The doctor sent her for a psychological evaluation, and Rosalie was diagnosed as a schizophrenic.

She spent time in a psychiatric hospital and was heavily medicated on antipsychotic drugs. She knew that she had to do and say whatever she needed to get out of that system, which is well meaning but inept at dealing with people who are psychic. Sadly, Rosalie met the same fate that many psychics have—she was told that she was crazy.

Even with model behavior, it took her six months to get out of the mental hospital where she was heavily drugged and endured several rounds of electroshock treatment. She told me later that the irony was the ECT treatments made her psychic ability much stronger. Her stay was very hard for her since the hospital was old, haunted, and full of negative energy. An angel and the spirit of her grandmother protected her during her stay in that horrible environment.

It's a testament to Rosalie's inner strength that she endured all of that at the tender age of seventeen. After she was released, her family watched her like a hawk for any recurrences of her "psychosis." She still had plenty of psychic experiences but never told anyone about them, including her husband and children, until she came to my psychic development class. Rosalie had taken Reiki and her psychic abilities were stronger than ever. At sixty years old, she was finally ready to embrace her gift and explore it, and work through the fear and trauma from the past.

It took a lot of inner work, healing sessions, and the support from her fellow students in her psychic class, but she got there. And, she was finally able to tell her husband and children about her gifts and what had happened to her as a young woman.

Sadly, Rosalie's experience used to be all too common for psychics, and it is one of the fears that many people need to work through to fully open to their gifts. Feeling crazy, going crazy, or being labeled as crazy are very real fears for psychics. There is a long and tragic history of psychics ending up in mental hospitals. There is a very blurry line between psychic and psychotic.

Sometimes psychics really *do* go a little crazy, if they have severe trauma that has never been healed. Plenty of psychics fear that once they open up, they will start seeing bad things or lose control of their abilities. This might happen if they don't have the proper training.

Here are some common fears people have about opening psychically:

- I'll start seeing horrible things.

- I've already had a bad experience; I don't want to open that door again.

- I won't be able to control what I see.

- I'll attract negative energy to me.

- I'll get possessed by a spirit and lose myself.

- It's like joining a cult.

- Other people will think I'm crazy.

- I'll go crazy.

- Someone told me that psychics practice witchcraft, and that's evil.

- It goes against my religion to talk to spirits.

- I'm afraid of the unknown.

Knowledge is powerful; the more you know about the spiritual worlds, the safer you are. It's like being street smart! You're far more apt to get into trouble if you don't learn anything and just bumble around in the dark.

Usually, the worst thing that happens is that spirit encounters scare us. This happens for two reasons. A paranormal encounter startles us when we aren't expecting it. The second reason is simply because it freaks us out when we have proof that spirits are real. That's a very earth-shaking event for most people, and it can really rock your world.

The first thing to do is to admit that you have a fear. Acknowledge it and see if you can find where it came from. You can release the fear by journaling about it, or talking it out with someone. Then, you can ask yourself if you have a good reason to be afraid. If so, take steps to make sure you are opening yourself in a safe manner and not doing the unsafe psychic activities that were discussed in chapter 2.

If you do psychic or healing work in a protected way, you won't go crazy or lose yourself. You must ground, clear, and protect yourself. And, you must work through your fear, or you'll be trying to open up your psychic ability with one foot on the gas and one foot on the brakes. This chapter provides information on psychic protection and how to work with your Reiki guides.

Psychic Protection Basics

If you want to make sure you are safe while you develop your psychic gifts, having a strong energy field and good energy management is a good place to start. (Check out chapter 4 for more information on energy management.) If your energy field is very strong, you won't have too much trouble with negative energy of any kind, whether from people or spirits. If you feel like you need more psychic protection, here are a few things that many psychics before you have found to be very helpful.

Sage and Incense

Aromatic smoke like sage, incense, and palo santo removes negative energy from an environment. This is why churches and temples burn incense. Aromatic smoke is fabulous at clearing our leftover human emotions, which is why we use it at the end of a healing session. It can also render a space uninviting to negative spirits. Here are some pointers for using sage:

- Use white sage, not culinary or cooking sage; they aren't the same thing.

- Sage your healing room before and after a session to clear the space.

- Sage your home regularly. (When my kids were little and everyone was fighting, I would sage the house, and they would all calm down quickly.)

- Sage can be useful to clear unwanted spirits at times, but mostly it's good for clearing leftover, residual human energy.

- Get sage spray if you can't burn it. Use this in hotel rooms, or anywhere else the energy feels funky.

If you don't like the smell of sage, which is very pungent, you can get sage that's mixed with other aromatics, like copal, lavender, or cedar. Palo santo is wood that has a sweet aroma that nearly everyone likes, and it has an uplifting energy. Frankincense and myrrh, available in incense form, are both great for space clearing. This is what churches traditionally use, and they're both great for dispelling sadness.

Salt

Salt is a powerful protectant and purifier. You can use any kind, from cheap table salt to Himalayan pink salt, which I favor. A salt lamp is one of the best things to have in bedrooms or healing rooms to keep the energy clear. Here are some ways I use salt:

- Put salt and baking soda in the tub with a few drops of essential oils for a bath that will clear your energy field. I prefer Epsom salt and lavender or sage oil for this.

- Put salt around your bed at night to keep away nightmares.

- Sprinkle salt around your house if spirits are passing through your house at night. You can salt your whole property, just be careful around plants, as it will kill them.

- Use a salt lamp in a child's room as a night-light. These are also very good for psychic and empathic children who feel spirits around them at night.

Running Water

Running water releases negative ions, which has a purifying effect on the environment and calming and healing effects on people. This is why we are drawn to the seaside, babbling brooks, and water-falls. It's also why feng shui practitioners use indoor fountains to bring good energy into living and working spaces.

Negative entities hate running water. They will run from it or jump off of you when you're around it. Running salt water is even better, so bathing in the surf of the ocean is one of the best things that you can do for your energy field. Here are some ways to use running water:

- Standing on a bridge over running water is a good way to clear your energy field.

- Have a water fountain with running water in your healing space or bedroom.

- Set up a fish tank with a filter that runs water. This is another good way to keep a child's room clear of spirits.

- Holy or blessed water is very handy to have around. It really works. You can get it from a church or temple, or bless some yourself using your Reiki.

HOW TO BLESS WATER

Hold a container of water in your hands. You can use water straight from the tap, or, better yet, put it in the sun or moonlight for a while before you bless it. Use your Reiki symbols to bless it. Each symbol will imbue the water with its own energy.

- *Chokurei* will charge the water for physical healing.

- *Seiheki* will charge the water for emotional energy.

- *Honshazeshonen* will clear up your thinking.

- *Dai Ko Myo* is for Divine energy. (Add this if you have Master Level attunement and know the symbol.)

- Use all the symbols for a very powerful combo!

- Charging the water in the sun will help you take action. Add the *Chokurei* symbol for this.

- Charging water in the moonlight will aid in emotional healing. Add the *Seiheki* symbol for more powerful emotional healing.

You can add a little of the blessed water to your tub, drink it, or put it in a spray bottle and spray it around.

Powerful Objects

Power objects can be anything from crystals and stones to crosses, rosaries, or other blessed objects. I love rosaries and have a whole collection of them from many different religions. I have blessed rosaries from Lourdes, St. Christopher medals, crosses, and mala beads from a temple in Thailand.

These objects have power and can be powerful protectors. Find some that resonate with you and wear them, or leave them around the house or in your car. I wear a blessed gold Celtic cross that I never take off. It's from Ireland and was blessed by an Irish priest. I wear it with a gold pendant of Our Lady of Fátima.

One of my friends wears a Wiccan pentagram blessed by a high priestess of her faith. Pentagrams were originally signs of the Goddess and a powerful protection symbol for women. Only recently, and quite sadly, have they been co-opted by Satanists as a symbol of the devil.

Any blessed power objects will work; just pick one that you resonate with and that fits with your faith tradition.

Tattoos

I think there can be great power in getting tattoos of protective symbols. I have a few myself, and they really work for me. Choose and place them wisely, for they have great power. I have seen people with powerful spells and incantations to the darkness, as well as gate-opening symbols tattooed on power spots on their bodies, such as at the seven chakra centers.

Make sure you research any symbol you like, and think long and hard about what it means and where you're going to put it before you tattoo it on yourself. Even a "good" symbol in the wrong place can have unintended outcomes. Be careful about using the Reiki symbols. You might not really want any particular symbol to always be in action on you or on one of your chakras. I worked with someone who had tattooed *Raku*, the symbol for opening, on her lower back, right on her second chakra. This was not good for her, as having that chakra wide open all the time can be problematic, especially considering it's the chakra for our sexuality and emotions. She couldn't figure out why she had become an emotional mess and a sex addict on top of that. She had to get a few more tattoos to balance herself back out again.

Q-Link

This is a device that will protect you from EMF (electromagnetic fields) radiation. Empaths are very sensitive to EMF radiation and should take precautions against it. EMF is generated by cell phones and other electronic devices, like computers, microwaves, and fluorescent lights. Too much EMF radiation will negatively impact your immune system, so it is especially bad for people with autoimmune problems.

The Q-Link, which can be worn as a necklace or a bracelet, will also greatly strengthen your energy field, and it can give an empath some peace when in psychically difficult situations. You can find it online.

Gemstones

Use gemstones in your healing spaces, wear them as jewelry, or carry them with you. Here are some that are great for psychic protection:

- Amethyst opens your third eye and can activate your dreams.

- Black onyx blocks negative influences.

- Black tourmaline is very grounding. It will keep you in your body.

- Clear quartz is my favorite one to use. It's very versatile. Use it to clear the energy field. You can also put it on a chakra to clear it.

- Labradorite protects against entities and psychic attack.

- Blue kyanite continually clears the energy field and never seems to lose its strength.

- Obsidian blocks negative energy and absorbs it.

Essential Oils and Flower Essences

I love working with essential oils! You can use them in your tub, on your body like a perfume, or in a diffuser. I use a diffuser in my room at night and in my healing room. Make sure you use the best-grade essential oil that you can find. I'm very picky about mine and

use only organic or wild-harvested essential oils. Here are some
essential oils that can be used for protection:

- Lavender to calm and bring peaceful, healing sleep at
  night

- Sage for space clearing

- Pine to clear your aura and dispel sadness

- Tangerine and grapefruit to clear entities and ghosts

- Clary sage for opening your third eye for clear seeing

- Galbanum for psychic protection and dispelling
  negativity

- Sandalwood to open the seventh chakra and to connect
  to your highest guides. (It's also wonderful for purifying
  energy.)

I also love working with flower essences, which can be very powerful and have no fragrance. My favorites are the Bach flower
essences, which are taken internally and can help stabilize our moods
and our energy levels. They are wonderful at helping us work through
specific issues that we are having.

Some flower essences are not for internal use. Instead, you use
them in your energy field and in the environment. I completely rely
on a company called Petaltones for these. I never leave home without
this company's space-clearing set. I have one set in my office, one at
home, and one that I carry in my purse, since I never know when I
will need these essences.

Prayer and Meditation

When in doubt, pray! Prayers come in many flavors and they're
all good. Say prayers that you love or are familiar with. When we
pray, we invoke the guides and angels around us. We invite them in
and we ask for Divine help and assistance.

Someone said that prayer is talking to God, and meditation is
listening for the answer. I love that and think it's true. When you feel

like you're not safe, pray. Start and end your day with prayer. It's one of the best things we can do to protect ourselves and keep our energy field healthy and clear.

Meditation is the best thing that you can do to increase your psychic ability. Meditation is good for everything. It's the best thing that I know of for better sleep and to decrease stress. And, it's the number one thing that you can do to open and develop your psychic abilities.

I love traditional sitting meditation, but I learned this as a child. My parents were hippies and took me to transcendental meditations. Since then, I have studied many different forms of sitting meditation. Meditation works for me, but it's very hard for most people without some practice and training.

There are many kinds of meditation, and they're all good. I use a breath method in which you consciously slow your breathing down and focus moving energy up your spine on the inhale, and then feel the breath on your upper lip as you exhale. If you want to start meditating (and I highly recommend that you do), here are some ways to begin:

- Try yoga. Yoga is a moving meditation. Moving the body shuts down the mind and can bring peace.

- Guided meditations are good for beginners, and there are many to choose from.

- If you really want to learn sitting meditation properly, take a class or join a group.

Working with Your Reiki Guides

Now that you have learned various ways to manage your energy and protect yourself psychically, it's time to meet your Reiki guides. Our Reiki guides are nonphysical beings whose goal is to help us while we are doing Reiki and in all aspects of our lives. Everyone has these guides, and they can be angels, teachers, departed relatives, or saints. (A nonhelpful or a neutral spirit being is called an *entity*. There is a huge variety of these kinds of beings, but we don't generally encounter them unless we go looking for trouble.)

Talking to your guides and listening to them is much easier than most people think. You have already been doing it your whole life, maybe without even knowing it. When most people consciously connect with their guides, they realize that it is something that they have been experiencing all along. It might be a familiar voice in their head, or a comforting presence.

Not everyone will see their guides. It's more likely that you will have a knowing feeling about them. Our connection with these beings is very natural but usually very subtle. It has been integrated into our unconscious lives from the time we're children. When we do figure out who our guides are and how they communicate, we often say something like "Oh that! That's been happening to me since I was a kid. It happens ten times a day, so I don't even think about it!"

As you work with them more frequently and get more comfortable, you'll have more contact with them. It takes practice and comfort on your part to get there. Here are some of the roles our guides fill for us:

Teachers: When you're studying Reiki, you will pull in guides whose job it is to teach. For example, when you are studying Reiki and healing, you might connect with a guide who specializes in that.

Event or Project Specific Guides: These guides show up for a certain event or time in your life. For example, while you're in school or traveling somewhere. You may have one while you're writing your dissertation or completing a big project at work. I had a guide who was just around me while I was pregnant; that was this guide's specialty.

People who are very creative will often feel like they're channeling the music they're playing, the art they're creating, or the words that they're writing. This type of guide is called a *muse*.

Emotional Guides and Counselors: These guides are connected to our emotional selves and will help us process our feelings and deal with big emotional events. They offer comfort and companionship.

Spiritual Directors: These guides will direct us on our spiritual path and are often connected to us for more than one lifetime. They really get the big picture! They arrive to help show us our path and will point us in the right direction when we're at a crossroads. They will also create situations that feel like obstacle courses so that we can reach our full potential in life.

Protectors and Guardians: These guides offer us their protection, usually energetically, by helping us with psychic self-defense and patching up our leaky aura. They can help with actual physical protection, too, especially with children. Think of them as bodyguards. Empaths always have a few of these around create protection around them in dicey environments.

Gatekeepers: These guides make connections for us across all the spiritual realms, and they hold open the gates and doors between worlds so that we can access different dimensions. If you're a medium, astral traveler, or dimension hopper, you really need to know about these guides. Mediums need them to keep out unwanted visitors and usher in specific spirits when needed.

Working Guides: These guides help us with whatever our life purpose is. If you're a healer, you will have guides who focus on assisting you while you're working. Same goes for any job that you do. If you're a nurse, for example, you'll have a guide who shows up when you're at work.

Healers: These guides work with us to help us heal from whatever is troubling us. They can help our minds, bodies, and spirits, but they seem to focus on helping us by doing a lot of energy work on us.

You probably have a whole team of guides when you do Reiki. You might have a teacher, a healer, and a guardian. Or, you might have one guide who is all of that for you. When you start working with your Reiki guides, you might meet a new one or meet one who you've been aware of for quite some time. Just know that they work with you and through you. It's also good to note that we can use prayer to ask different guides to be present for us.

Types of Guides

Distinct from the roles they play, there are many different types of guides—perhaps an infinite variety. You could have a healer guide who's an angel, a dead relative, or a being of pure energy. Here are some of the types of guides.

ANGELS

Angels are often what people think of when they consider their guides. Angels are nonhuman beings of light. They have never been human and never will be, so it's not like you die and become an angel.

I notice that some people are "angel people" who attract angels around them. You will know if you're an angel person. Empaths often love angels and attract them as spirit guides. Everyone has a different experience of the angels. To me, they never look human. I see them as huge columns of light, or sometimes balls of light. They are wonderful guides and have extraordinary love and patience for humanity.

ANCESTOR GUIDES

Ancestor guides are the souls of our loved ones who have crossed over and help us. Some people have a huge connection to their beloved ancestors, whereas others don't. If you come from a tight-knit family, or had one special relative who was a deep soul mate to you when he or she was alive, then you might have some ancestor guides on your team.

These are easy guides to work with, since we're not usually afraid of them. Just a little forewarning: dying doesn't always change some-one's personality. You should think about whose advice you're taking. I've seen plenty of wonderful, kind, and well-meaning ancestor guides, and quite a few nosy, bossy ones.

SOUL FAMILY GUIDES

These guides are part of our *soul family*, rather than our actual family. They're like soul mates. We never have just one soul mate! Instead, we have a group or a tribe. We usually see them in human form, and often they'll appear in a form that we remember them, in having another life. They are very easy to work with and sometimes are the first guides that we encounter because they're so familiar and already loved. We trust them right away.

MASTERS, SAINTS, AND PROPHETS

These are souls who used to be human but have evolved beyond the cycle of incarnation. They stay around to help the rest of us evolve. Examples of the masters include Jesus, Mary, Buddha, and Kwan Yin.

They are very powerful guides to work with and almost all of us are aligned with one of these as our spiritual teacher. There are plenty of them around who have never had books written about them, or religions formed around them, but are wonderful guides all the same. They are very knowing and compassionate about the human experience.

POWER ANIMALS

These are the energy and essences of animals. They are very pure and simple energies and help us in many ways. People who have an interest in shamanism or who are deep nature lovers will often access power animals. Power animals act as guards and bring us pure energy frequencies. For example, a lion may give you the energy of courage and strength, and a dolphin may give you the pure energy of joy and playfulness.

EARTH SPIRITS

These are the spiritual essences of the natural world, including plant spirits and elementals. *Elementals* are spirits who represent the four elements of earth, air, fire, and water. Other earth spirits are the spirits of rocks, trees, mountains, rivers, lakes, and forests.

There are also fairy beings. Some of these beings are helpful to humanity, and some are not. I find them tricky, a bit mercurial in nature, and prone to trickster-type behaviors. If you're a friend to the fairy folk, these beings will be devoted and protective of you. If you aren't, and you encounter them, they might trick you, trip you up, or be otherwise generally mischievous. Hardcore gardeners and nature lovers, you might be fairy folk!

PURE ENERGY BEINGS

These beings are from many different places and serve many different purposes. The main characteristic of these beings is that they're not from planet earth. They're also not human, but neither are they angelic or fairy beings. They can be classified as multidimensional beings, and there is an infinite variety of them. They can look like anything but often appear as balls of light, commonly called *orbs*. They are one of the most common types of guides, and they are always very high frequency.

As I said, you may well have a combination of these guides, and over time you will come to know all the guides who work with you. As we work with our guides and get to know them, it's important to remember some basic ground rules.

Ground Rules for Working with Your Guides

When we're working with our guides, it's good to keep these essential guidelines in mind. The first rule is that our guides cannot and will not interfere with our free will or take away a lesson or an experience that we need for our growth and evolution. They are here to help us with our spiritual evolution, but it is not in their nature to live life for us, or to take away our choices and lessons.

Expecting them to totally fix things for you is like asking your teacher to do your homework. You won't learn anything that way. I have seen people ask their guides to take away their life lessons because they are too painful. That is not something they can do. They can advise, cheer us on, and assist from the sidelines. They might help you connect to the right healer so that you can have the help you need to work through something. They might inspire you to find a way to help yourself, or give you a moment of grace to regain your faith.

It's too much to expect your guides to make every decision for you. Free will is the major universal law that we live under, and so our guides will never interfere with our choices. They will advise, offer solutions, and point out the outcomes of our potential choices. They will be cheerleaders, comforters, protectors, and companions, but they won't bail you out of your karma or lessons. They're focused on our maximum growth potential, not doing our work for us.

There is a little wiggle room here for the occasional miracle, when our guides will step in to truly save us. I see this most often when we're in danger and it won't help us to die at that moment because we haven't finished what we came here to do. So, they might step in to help in extreme moments.

Our guides also can't and won't interfere with the free will of other people. That would be black magic. There are exceptions to this, as with small children. You might ask your guides to watch over your kids, for example, and they'll do what they can. But, don't expect them to keep your boyfriend from breaking up with you, if that's what he chooses to do. Watch your agenda.

HANDS-ON OR HANDS-OFF GUIDANCE

Some people have a very tight connection to their guides and feel them in every moment. These are what I call the *hands-on* guides. They're with us every step of the way! This is how my guides are; they're very bossy and direct with me and always have been. My joke is, "I just show up and do what I'm told." It works for me. In exchange, I receive a constant stream of information from them all. Since I work as a professional psychic, it's all good.

Other people don't want or need that, so their guides are more *hands-off.* I notice that some people prefer figuring out stuff all by themselves and hate to be told what to do. If that describes you, your guides will be around but will stay out of your hair unless you specifically ask for help.

CONTACTING YOUR GUIDES

Working with your Reiki guides is about building a relationship. It happens slowly over time. The more you pay attention and just let this special relationship flow, the more you will be aware of.

Doing frequent mediation, prayer, or spiritual practice will give your guides an opportunity to communicate with you. One of the things that our guides complain about the most is that we don't create an open listening space for them. Our lives and our minds are so crowded. We're too busy and noisy to listen to our own inner guidance and theirs.

One of the best things you can do to build the relationship with you guides is to have a regular time dedicated to just listening and receiving information. This can be when you're alone in the woods, during prayer or meditation, or just on your daily walk. Doing this regularly is the easiest way to deepen your relationship with your guides.

Although we're talking about your Reiki guides, chances are very good that these guides want to work with you in the whole of your life, not just while you're doing Reiki. Cultivating a relationship with them can have a huge and beneficial impact on your entire life.

ALPHA STATE

We need to go into a mildly altered state of consciousness to contact our guides. We can learn to change our brain-wave frequency to the alpha wave, which is a very light trance state. When we're totally conscious and awake, our brain is in the beta brain-wave state. This is highly logical and analytical, but not at all intuitive.

The alpha brain-wave is where all psychic ability, intuition, and creativity come from. Good psychics and shamans learn how to shift their brain states at will to access deeper levels of consciousness. Shamans use things like drumming, dancing, and sound toning to shift states. Meditators use their meditation techniques and breath practices to do it. Yogis use yoga asanas and pranayama to shift into an alpha state.

Any kind of spiritual practice will do it, or anything that is mildly boring and repetitive, like driving, mowing the lawn, or washing the dishes. The alpha brain-wave is very soothing, relaxing, and creative. We connect with our guides and get intuitive hits, creative inspirations, and problem-solving insights in this state.

We have all had the experience of puzzling over some difficult problem only to finally give up on it to go walk the dog, weed the garden, or fold the laundry. The next thing you know, the answer magically pops into your mind, as soon as you stopped thinking about it!

Things that will get you into a receptive state:

- Prayer or meditation

- Journal writing

- Playing with tarot cards or a pendulum

- Taking a walk in nature

- Relaxing in the tub

- Yoga, tai chi, or qigong

- Driving a car

- Doing the dishes, taking a shower, or working in the garden

- Sitting on the beach, staring at the ocean, or staring into a fire

- Chanting or singing

- Getting or giving energy work

- Sleeping and dreaming

- Engaging in a creative activity

You will strengthen your connection to your guides when you make space to listen to what they are saying.

THE INVISIBLE HANDS

It's usually around the time that you really connect to your Reiki guides that your Reiki clients will experience the phenomenon of the "invisible hands." I remember the first time this happened to me; I was lying on the table with my eyes covered by an eye pillow. My Reiki practitioner was working on my feet, but I could feel someone else's hands on my head. I was confused because I hadn't heard anyone else come into the room. But, both sets of hands felt the same. I could feel how hot the second pair of hands were!

When the session was over, I eagerly took off my eye pillow to see who had joined us in the session. To my surprise, no one was there but my practitioner. It was just she and I in the room, but I had felt two sets of hands on me. That's when she explained the invisible hands to me. This other set of hands belonged to her Reiki guide who was there in the session with us. It was so incredibly concrete. I could feel heat, pressure, and the sensation of another pair of hands on me. If you practice Reiki enough, sooner or later you or one of your clients will have this experience.

GETTING CONFIRMATION

When we first start working consciously with our guides, it's important to get confirmation from them that they are who they say they are. Real guides would never expect you to just take their word for who they are without proof of some kind. You can tell your guides what kind of proof you'd prefer, but usually they'll do something in the real world to help you know that they're around. It's common for people to ask for things like pennies or feathers to show up as proof.

When we ask for proof, our guides will shower us with signs and omens. We need to be on the lookout for them, though, or we might miss them. Angels seem particularly fond of pennies and feathers, which is why so many people associate the two. A student of mine challenged her guides to prove they were real, as she was very skeptical about the whole thing. She got a little angry about it and really put her foot down. The moment she demanded that they show her a sign, a big white feather floated down from the sky and landed on the ground right in front of her. She's been a believer ever since. She told me the feather looked like it could be an angel's.

Another one of my students picked a hard sign, or so she thought. She wanted to be shown a giraffe as a sign, knowing that living in the suburbs of Boston she was not likely to see one just walking down the street. That afternoon, her son came off the school bus with a friend from school. The friend was wearing a shirt that had a big giraffe on it. She had to laugh, knowing that was her sign.

This kind of stuff is fun, so don't be afraid to be a little playful about it. It's fine to have a little fun with your guides!

THE ART OF DISCERNMENT

What do we do when we have an experience with a spirit who makes us uncomfortable? The chances are good that at some point in developing your psychic abilities, you will encounter this. Discernment is a psychic skill that helps you know what kind of spirit you're dealing with. The most basic form of discernment is something that all of us use, all the time, without even thinking about it. We do this every time we meet someone new. We immediately unconsciously categorize people into three distinct groups.

- Good and benevolent

- Neutral

- Bad, yucky, or evil

This is a deep kind of intuitive knowing; we instinctively know which category someone falls into. It might be a sensation in your body, like a queasy stomach. Or, it could be a good or bad feeling or a sense of knowing. The information can come along any of your psychic channels, but, one way or another, you are going to know if you feel good, neutral, or yucky.

This is the same kind of discernment that you should be using when you encounter a new spirit. Let's say you wake up in the middle of the night and feel the presence of a spirit in your room. This is a very common psychic experience that nearly every psychic has experienced. Very likely the first thing that will happen is that you will feel startled. That's perfectly normal, and no doubt it would also startle you to find an unexpected living person in your room at night too. Once you get over being startled, you'll want to notice how you *feel.*

- If you feel good, it's a beneficial spirit. You'll feel uplifted, light, and happy. Check in with your body. Your belly will tell you. These are benevolent guides and are very good to work with.

- You might feel neutral—neither good nor bad, just in the middle. If so, then you've attracted a neutral spirit to yourself. They are usually just curious, and although they aren't harmful, it's best to move them along.

- If you feel very frightened or get a feeling of dread or terror, you have attracted a negative spirit, which we call "entities." These spirits are trouble and you need to get rid of them.

Once you know what kind of spirit you are dealing with, you can decide what to do about it. Work with the good ones, politely move along the neutral ones, and get rid of the bad ones.

SPIRIT, BE GONE!

If you do encounter a spirit who makes you uncomfortable, here is what you can do to help it move along. I treat spirits a lot like I treat people. It's good to give them the benefit of the doubt and politely ask them to leave, just as I would any person. Most of the time, being polite and asking them to move along works very well. Sometimes they are surprised that you can sense them, and they didn't know they were bothering you. At this point, it's not necessary to break into a full exorcism. Just politely ask them to leave.

One of my friends has a daughter who is very psychic and has strong mediumship abilities. Her daughter said that the spirits kept her up at night and bothered her so she couldn't sleep. She learned how to politely ask them to leave, because she needed her sleep, and to tell them that she would talk to them all in the morning. Eventually, she put a sign on her door listing her "office hours" and a request not to be bothered at night.

Sometimes it isn't enough to simply ask them to leave, and we must raise the bar. This is where we *demand* that they leave.

Remember that you are the powerful one. Spirits, ghosts, entities, and even guides have very little power in this dimension. Stomp your foot, point your finger, and use your "bad dog" voice. And, really mean it! Demand that they leave and leave for good. Often this does the trick, just as it would with most people.

If *that* doesn't work, then you have to call on a higher power: "In the name of Jesus Christ, *I demand* that you leave now!" This almost always works. You can use any deity of your choice here. Archangel Michael is always a good pick, and Jesus is probably the most famous exorcist ever. But, choose whomever you resonate with. This is the spiritual equivalent of calling the cops. Let a higher power do the heavy lifting; it's better for you.

In some cases, this won't work either. This is when you would call in a professional for help. You might ask a priest to do a house blessing or call in a feng shui practitioner who will also do a blessing for you. There are also psychics and healers who specialize in house clearings. Sometimes paranormal groups will do this, but make sure to engage groups that will do a clearing, otherwise it could make your situation worse.

People are much more comfortable working with their guides when they know that they're in charge and in control. Working with your guides should be easy, pleasant, and natural, not something that scares you. So, have a little fun with it!

❀ Cheryl's Story ❀
Mother Mary Is My Guide

I was nervous about working with my Reiki guides. I grew up in a very religious family, so I was taught that speaking to spirits was wrong. I never thought of myself as psychic, so I was nervous and skeptical. When I first did the meditation, I didn't see much. I saw colors, like when you see light shining through a stained-glass window. But, it did feel good. I got the feeling of a woman who was kind and compassionate. The answers popped into my head; I just knew.

*My guide said her name was Mary, and she was here to help
me heal myself and other people, and that she was all about love.*

*After a while, I felt her more and more often when I was
doing Reiki sessions. I would see that colored light behind my
eyes, and I knew that she was there. In the Reiki sessions, she
would sometimes put her hands on mine, or tell me what to do,
where to move next, and how long to stay there. She said simple
but profound things, like "This person is really sad and they need
to cry. Do the heart sandwich for a long time until they can
release it." So, I did that and my client cried on the table and felt
a lot better afterward.*

*Mary was always right, and after a while I relaxed because it
just felt so natural and easy. I wondered how I was ever scared of
her. She would also come to me in my meditations and dreams
and tell me things about my own life.*

*My clients would say they felt another pair of hands when I
was working, which I thought was so cool. I wondered who she
was, so I asked her. She laughed and said, "Mary, as in Mother
Mary." I couldn't believe it at the time, but I had been talking to
her and praying to her since I was a child. Now, I just roll with it,
because it works and makes me and my clients feel better. I don't
think the church would mind so much since it's her, so I feel safe.*

Meet Your Reiki Guides

Now that we have explored the concept of your Reiki guides, it's
time to have your own experience with them. Try this exercise with
an open mind and do your best to release your expectations about
what you think might or should happen. Just relax and allow whatever is unfolding to be there without judgment. Our guides tend to
make this first contact gentle, especially if you are nervous about it.
The last thing your guides want to do is to scare you.

Do this mediation often. As you get used to the concepts and the
presence of your guides, chances are good that you will have some
interesting experiences with them. Remember that these are relationships, and it takes time to build any kind of relationship.

MEET YOUR REIKI GUIDES MEDITATION

Find a quiet place, and sit in a chair with your feet on the floor. Take a few deep breaths to center yourself in your body.

Inhale deeply and breathe light into the top of your head. This opens the crown chakra. Fill your whole body with light, bringing it into your heart and belly with each in-breath.

Exhale down your legs and spine, releasing down into the earth any thoughts or emotions that you're holding. Whatever you're holding on to for yourself or other people, you can now let it go, down into the ground. This grounds you and reconnects you to the earth.

The exhale breath is a clearing breath. Release all that you're carrying that no longer serves you.

With each deep inhale, continue to bathe your whole body in light. This is a filling breath that replaces your lost energy.

You now should feel solidly grounded to the earth. Your energy field has been cleared. Gently bring awareness to your heart area, as you begin the Reiki breath.

Imagine your crown chakra opening as you inhale deeply, breathing light in through the top of your head. Now exhale down your spine to the ground and down into the earth.

Again, inhale deeply, breathing up the front of your body into your heart. Fill up your heart with your cleansing breath until it overflows.

As you exhale, let the overflow of energy from your heart move down your arms and into your hands. Be aware of the warmth building in your hands as the Reiki energy activates.

As you feel the Reiki energy flow through you, call in your guides. Give them your permission to join you.

Taking a deep breath, state, "I ask that my Reiki guides come forward and be here with me now."

Stilling your mind, continue to breathe deeply, and patiently stay open to any insights. Consciously release any expectations. Stay open to any colors, feelings of another's presence, or anything you hear or see in your mind's eye. You might feel something in your body, with your emotions, or with your knowing. Allow this experience to unfold in whatever way it wishes to.

Ask your guides these questions:

- What is your name?

- What is your purpose for working with me?

- What is the best way for me to contact you? How do you send me messages?

- Is there anything you want to tell me or that I need to know?

Feel free to ask any questions you have about anything on your mind now. Listen for your answers. You may hear them, feel them, or have a knowing. Let the information come to you in whatever form it chooses. There is no wrong way to receive guidance.

When you have finished talking to your guides, thank them for their service. You can reach them anytime you wish by using this meditation. Ground any excess energy you may have by breathing it down the grounding cord and into the earth. If you feel light-headed or dizzy, exhale deeply and come back into your body. Push your feet into the floor and wiggle your toes and fingers. When you feel ready, slowly open your eyes and come back to full awareness.

The Takeaway

In this chapter, I covered a lot of ground for how to effectively and joyfully work with your spirit guides. Most people need to begin by addressing and cleaning up any fear they have of psychic work, since it is very hard to open to your guides if you are still afraid. It's also important to learn some psychic self-defense techniques so that we can be safe when we are working with our guides. The psychic protection basics I covered included things like using blessed water and how to use salt to purify. I covered a lot of other ways to protect yourself, like using essential oils and flower essences, gemstones and crystals, and blessed objects.

I also outlined all the different types of guides you might encounter, which is important to understand since most of us have a team of guides. It's nice to know who our team is and how to best receive information from them. Connecting with our guides is about practicing and remembering that we are cultivating a relationship with them. It's important to ask for confirmation, so we know our guides are legitimate. It's equally important to feel confident enough to ask spirits to move along if we don't feel comfortable with their presence. Learning to work directly with your guides is one the most fun and rewarding aspects of Psychic Reiki, and I know you are off on a grand adventure.

In the epilogue, we are going to take a peek into what awaits you at Reiki Level 3, which we also call the Master Level. It's a very exciting and joyful level to study, and I encourage you all to continue on to this level of Reiki. At Reiki Level 3, we go deeply into how to do spiritual-healing work as well as how to do the attunements. It's wonderful to learn how to do attunements, which are part of the magic of Reiki Level 3.

Reiki Level 3

It's difficult to try and condense all the wonderful power of Reiki Level 3 into an epilogue, but I want to encourage you to continue your Reiki training and move into Reiki Level 3 if you haven't already. If you are already a Reiki Master, then I encourage to continue to study your Reiki skills. I will go back to what I said in the very beginning of this book—the world needs all the healers it can get!

With Reiki Level 3, you will receive your Master Level attunement. There is something very joyful about this attunement. The Level 1 and 2 attunements tend to bring up things that need healing, so although they are very powerful and life changing, they can also bring about a healing crisis. The Reiki Level 3 attunement is much more likely to bring a more permanent state of joy with it. Many Reiki practitioners report that they feel noticeably lighter, happier, and more joyful, and that this state becomes their new baseline of happiness. I think that is wonderful and worth pursuing on its own merits.

At the Reiki Master Level, we learn the Master Symbols, which allow us to do the attunements and bring in the power of spiritual healing. *Spiritual healing* is addressing wounds that occur at the spiritual level, such as past-life issues, the spiritual foundations of our mental and physical health, and our soul-level contracts with people.

The Reiki Master Level symbols are powerful and very healing, and most people fall in love with them. The master symbol *Dikomyo* means "align with the Divine," and it helps us to do that, which is why working with this symbol brings about such a state of peace and joy.

You will also learn how to give attunements to other people. It's a fabulous way to share the Reiki love. Because the attunements themselves are so healing, I encourage you to practice the attunements on anyone you can. Naturally, you need to be working with a Reiki Master to receive your Master Level attunement. Find a teacher whom you resonate with, and study hard. There is a deeper spiritual practice that goes with the Master Level training. This is an excellent time to level up your spiritual practice and really commit to something like a daily yoga or a meditation routine, so that you can continue to strengthen those spiritual muscles.

Let's talk about the word "master." Some people don't feel comfortable progressing at this level since they don't yet feel like a master. It's good to be humble about your Reiki practice, but don't let that stand in your way of continuing to learn. The concept of a Reiki Master is something that we earn and step into over a long period of time. True Reiki Masters are the ones who keep studying, learning, and doing many Reiki sessions. If we truly want to earn the title Reiki Master we must continue to learn new skills, practice Reiki, and deepen and commit to a spiritual practice. We are Reiki Masters, and we are also continuing to move down the path to more and more mastery.

Reiki teachers all have different rules about how long you should study at Reiki Level 2 before you can take your Reiki Master training. Some people have studied Reiki Level 2 for a year or so, and some learn Reiki Levels 1, 2, and 3 very quickly together. Let your intuition guide you about how long you need at each level before you progress.

Becoming a Reiki Master reminds me of how I felt when I got my black belt in Okinawan Goju-Ryu karate. Earning a black belt is like becoming a Reiki Master, but I was surprised when I went to my first black belt class. I thought I had arrived and that I had reached the goal, the endgame of my training. However, I found that the senior students were doing new forms and breaking down each move, really studying its application. There was so much more to learn that I had never even imagined was possible.

Rather than feeling puffed up about my achievement, I felt humbled and awestruck. The senior-level black belts informed me that the belt was there to keep your pants up and that was about it. They explained that in the past, the belt had been there to keep your uniform tidy, and it turned black over time due to sweat and hard work.

If you study Reiki this way, you will feel like a master before you know it. With the Reiki Master Level, you also learn deeper spiritual-healing techniques. This is when you would learn past-life healing techniques and perceive how people's past lives are still affecting them in this life. Past-life work is exciting and interesting, and it perfectly blends spiritual healing with your increased psychic abilities.

At Reiki Level 3, your psychic abilities will weave seamlessly into your healing sessions, so that it all becomes one and it's hard to separate out what is Reiki and what is psychic ability. This is also part of mastering this level of Reiki. You may also become aware of where your clients need spiritual healing. It might be past-life events that have not fully been processed and are bleeding over into this life. It also might be the spiritual roots of mental health and physical issues. Sometimes our clients have deep pain and problems that have roots in past lives. As healers, we might have difficulty finding the root cause unless we are able to do this level of spiritual healing.

Spiritual healing might also include helping people work through the lingering energetic connections we have with relationships that have ended. Reiki Masters will see these energy cords that connect us in unhealthy ways in our relationships. Looking at the spiritual contracts between people and learning to do cord cutting is a powerful way that you can help your clients. It brings almost instant relief to painful relationships.

Many people at the Reiki Master Level will learn how to do psychic surgery. It's a very useful technique that we might use to heal a ripped chakra, "sew" up a torn aura, and even remove strange objects that we can feel energetically embedded into people's energy fields. For example, I recently did a session on someone who had gone through a painful breakup. She was still very sad and depressed about it, weeping throughout the session even though she knew it was not a healthy relationship for her. Once she was on the table, I had a vision of a knife stuck in the back of her heart. I asked her about it. She said she felt that way because there had been a huge betrayal in the relationship. I gently removed this energetic knife and had to sew up her leaking heart chakra. It was really a broken heart. It felt like a very karmic relationship, so it was important to explore the soul contract she had with this person. I could see a past life where she had been this person's mother, and she still felt like she had to mother and protect him, despite his tendencies toward self-destructive behavior.

She was relieved to learn about this dynamic. It helped explain her feelings toward him and why he might not be a good pick for a romantic partner. We finished the session with a cord cutting, which helped release the unhealthy desire she had to save, fix, and rescue him and offered some closure for her.

You can see from this example how all those spiritual issues were woven together to create a painful block for her. The Reiki Master Level is all about being able to perceive these connections and then using these advanced healing techniques to help the client release a wound at the spiritual level. It's powerful stuff! At this level, it's also very good to learn about how to handle clients who have deeper trauma, as many of your clients will. People who have unhealed traumas are drawn to all kinds of healing work and may well seek out energy healings, as well as counseling and other methods. More and more Reiki practitioners are being called on to help people who have severe trauma, and working with these people is something that you need training for as a Reiki Master. It's a horrible feeling to be in the middle of a Reiki session and have a client reveal a deep trauma and not know how to handle it. Sadly, this happens all too frequently. Becoming skilled in how to assist someone who is healing from a trauma is critical training for Reiki Masters. We also need to learn how to hold on to ourselves in those sessions, because they can be difficult to witness. When we ourselves are traumatized by hearing the story of a client's trauma, it is called *secondary trauma*. We need to learn how to care for ourselves when that happens.

The last and maybe most important piece of Reiki Master training is to find a way to bring your Reiki out into the world. For some, it's a practice with clients, which is how I do it. For some, their Reiki practice might be part-time, something done out of love on their days off. Other people are called to volunteering. Reiki Masters volunteer in hospitals, nursing homes, and hospice centers. They hold babies in neonatal wards or they are nurses who give the blessing of Reiki every time they touch a patient.

Reiki is a fabulous additive for anyone who works hands-on with others. Hairdressers, massage therapists, and physical therapists greatly benefit from adding Reiki to their toolkits. Reiki blends so nicely with other healing modalities that energy and body workers can use it along with their other modalities.

It's an important part of your Reiki journey to understand where Reiki is calling you to use it in the world, and then to do so. Perhaps you are called to work with animals or children. Maybe it's lots of "Kitchen Table Reiki" with your friends and family. Or, maybe you are drawn to using long-distance Reiki for the upsets and disasters that are on the news. Reiki is like a prayer that can be a powerful healing agent on a global level. Don't underestimate the power of this, even though it might seem ordinary and humble.

Your guides will send you "clients" of all kinds and in all ways, when you are open to it. It might be a friend or family member in need. It might be a client paying for a session or a person you see in need in your community. It might be a public tragedy, or a small, unnoticed interaction with the person standing behind you in a checkout line. When we have the spirit of Reiki, it moves through us any way it can, and that is a beautiful thing.

It has been my honor and privilege to be one of your Reiki teachers, and I wish you wonderful, healing experiences as your Reiki journey continues. Let us conclude with the wisdom of Usui Sensei and the Reiki principles:

Just for today do not worry.

Just for today do not anger.

Honor your parents, teachers, and elders.

Earn your living honestly.

Show gratitude to everything.

Reiki for Animals
by Sharon Wilsie

Animals need special considerations when we do Reiki. I want to take a moment to honor Sharon Wilsie, one of my own Reiki teachers and an expert in working with animals. The following comprises Sharon's experience and tips on treating animals with Reiki.

Animals receive Reiki on different levels than humans do. They do not have preconceived notions about energy work, so when you begin to perform Reiki on them, they respond directly to the experience they are having with you. Occasionally, when animals first begin to sense the shift in energy, they become nervous about it. Animals are much more present to what is happening directly in their environment than humans tend to be, which can be a rewarding experience for the people who are working on them.

To begin working on an animal, it's important to make sure you have had a proper introduction, *especially* if you're not accustomed to the species you are working on. If, for instance, you were working on a wounded owl at a sanctuary, you would want to introduce yourself, in your mind and in your actions, as if the animal were a person. It can be helpful to speak out loud, as our spoken words create tiny micromovements in our facial and body languages. Animals are highly attuned to reading energy and intention through sound and movement. Animals have advanced proprioceptive awareness, which means they study these micromovements to discern our intentions and purpose.

Animals are masters in body language, which is why you can't lie to them! They will see it if you are scared, nervous, or in any way dissociated. The brilliant thing about animals is that you don't have to be completely fearless or strong; if you're honest about it, they will feel comfortable with you. They hate dishonesty because to them it feels like your insides don't match your outsides, and this incongruence makes them nervous about your real intentions. Simply tell animals how you feel about working on them, and what your intentions really are, including any reservations you may have, and ask them to be forgiving of your weaknesses.

I recently worked on a squirrel that had been stunned by running into my car, even though I had tried to swerve out of the way. After pulling over to the side of the road and moving the squirrel to the woods, I began to do gentle Reiki on him. I began with his third eye, since he was in shock. Combining a soothing stroking motion with my fingers on his head, I sent energy to his head to allow him to make the next step without fear. I thought he might die in my hands and was prepared for this, and I told him he was safe and it was okay. I would be there for his transition.

His breathing slowed and he blinked, then he began licking his lips. This is always a good sign that the animal is shifting in his experience. I gently stroked down his spine and sent Reiki through my fingertips as I did. I was feeling for injuries energetically, and I was surprised to discover that I did not detect any.

Why, then, was he not moving his legs? I lifted his legs, sending Reiki up and down each leg, and finally I pulled the stress of the accident out of his tail with three consecutive gentle tugs. Immediately, he wanted to get up, so I backed off. He leapt to his feet and then scurried up a tree!

The primary difference in doing Reiki on an animal versus doing a human Reiki session is that animals are in a more available flow of moving energy. When doing a healing session on humans, one often runs into blocked energy or blocked chakras. There are numerous reasons why people become blocked, but because of that the practitioner needs to take the time to work out that stuck energy and try to get it flowing again. Most often, animals are not blocked anywhere, unless there has been a serious trauma or injury that has caused a temporary break in the flow. Even where there are emotional issues, overall the animal will not be completely blocked off.

It's important to remember to move faster than you normally would on a person, and to follow the flow from point to point rather than lingering on a specific spot too long. While it's true that animals have the same chakra system that we have, after performing a scan of each chakra, the practitioner is advised to move down all the limbs and out the tail before settling on the spots that stand out as needing more attention. You can figure out the spots that need more healing energy by learning to sense when a spot makes you feel out of breath, tense, or clamped down. You may even feel a sudden twinge or ache yourself.

Your own body is the best device to trust when determining the healing needs of the animal. You will find yourself wanting to take a big breath and relax when the animal is truly receiving the healing. Some animals will receive a full healing in only a few minutes. Some learn to love Reiki and will seek out longer sessions. My cats will request that I place my hands on parts of their body as they lounge in my lap.

I have had various pets come down with serious life-threatening illnesses that the vet believed they would die from. Whether it was a horse in full colic, a dog that got poisoned, or a cat with a terrible infection, when I did Reiki on them they got relief. Sometimes I would work through the night, applying dozens of power sessions in which I would find the *spot*, and the animal would lean into it and begin to breathe deeply.

In all these cases, I was willing to stay up all night and treat the beloved pet in what I call a *power session*, which means I combine deep breathing and my own higher consciousness through the crown chakra, and channel the power of healing through my own altered state of awareness. Be careful, though; in serious cases, if your emotions are running too high, they will not help the animal heal.

What is essential is to maintain an altered state of higher awareness during the session and attempt to contact the animal's higher self. When we do Reiki, we go into an altered state of consciousness ourselves, and this helps us access our own higher awareness, which is the wisdom of our higher self. This is not as hard as you might think. Animals are more of an open book than we are, and their higher self is usually quite interested in talking to our higher self.

Do not confuse a pet's higher self with its core personality. A cat has a cat's brain and a cat's concerns. It will scratch you from its lower self, which may be feeling fear or pain, even as the higher self is talking about transcended awareness. Animals have an animal's instincts and a *small* self, along with their wisdom and higher self, just like us. If you see the animal beginning to squirm in the middle of a treatment, then adjust your work, or even stop. They know when they have had enough, so trust them.

When one of my cats contracted the feline flu, she got so dehydrated that her kidneys started to shut down. The vet thought she would die, so I asked to just take her home with the appropriate medicine and a bag of IV fluids. I have vet-tech training, so administering medications to animals is comfortable for me, and I would rather run fluids at home where I can also run a steady stream of Reiki.

My kitty flopped on her side and allowed me to sandwich her belly and back with my hands. We snuggled up in my bed for a long night, and by the morning she was requesting food, and to use the litter box. By the end of that day, she was lying in her favorite sunny spot, and within three days she was back to normal. The vet tested her kidney functions and could not find a trace of the shutdown. She had excellent chemistry levels, and all her blood work was fine!

I have administered Reiki to chickens, horses, donkeys, ducks, peacocks, dogs, cats, parrots, bunnies, wild critters that I rescued from my cats' mouths, and even toads, snakes, and fish. In all cases, the animals become very still, and then they want to go off by themselves for a bit. After a short time, they are usually "shaking it off" and starting to look healthy again. Because animals are normally open and in the flow of their life force, it doesn't take much to reestablish homeostasis.

Consider that animals are almost always in a state of being that naturally seeks to rebalance inner harmony. Mother Nature is whispering, and they are listening to her loud and clear. All we need to do is gently nudge them in the right direction when something has become overwhelming for them, such as in the case of abuse.

If you have a rescued animal you are trying to work on, you will want to avoid talking about its history while in its presence, unless to do so is to validate its feelings about the abuse from a strong place of believing in its ability to overcome. Animals resent having their stories become a source of interesting drama for humans to focus on, and they really do not appreciate having to relive the same trauma over again every time their caregiver tells the story to someone new. Animals are very willing to be in the here and now and to let go of their memories of a troubled past. Although they may exhibit the typical hypersensitivity that anyone experiencing PTSD will have, they are quite willing to believe in a new day.

When working with a traumatized animal, tell it out loud that it is safe now, and expect it to have decent manners and boundaries like any other animal is expected to have when it's with you. Tiptoeing around an abused animal makes it feel as if something must be wrong with it, and this makes it feel worse.

In the animal kingdom, a cat will treat an abused cat like any other cat; a dog will treat an abused dog like any other dog. The other animals will not pander to a nervous animal, because they want the delicate one to feel like it is at home now, just one of the pack, and that everything is okay. This doesn't mean that you should be loud, gruff, or demanding. Telling the animal you believe in its power to overcome will have a much better outcome than assuming it's damaged goods forever.

I have worked extensively for thirty years with animals from all circumstances. I once worked with a cat who had to have skin grafts over half of her body due to having been severely abused. We nick-named her "Franken-kitty" to keep the energy light around her, and we allowed her free range of the house. We encouraged her not to hide under the bed and made her a special cat tree all her own, from which she had the vantage point to oversee the whole house. In only a month, she was pushing the other cats out of the way around food and was standing up for herself to have "lap rights" when we watched TV. Along with the daily Reiki treatments, we told her repeatedly what an amazing, strong being she was. Frank moved on to a loving home, where she ruled the roost.

How to Facilitate an Animal Reiki Treatment

Become very quiet on the inside, calm your emotions, and go into an altered state. Call in your guides to assist, but also call in the animal's guides and the animal's higher self to talk to you. As you approach the pet, tell it out loud exactly what your intentions are. Extend your knuckles to its nose, which is a universal animal "handshake" that makes you seem safe.

As you begin your first treatment, start with the pet's third eye, and press down on this spot with a strong exhaled breath. Draw your fingers down its nose area and flick the tension out and away from its third eye. Most animals really love this and will be onboard with whatever you want to do after.

Now resume with your fingers or the cup of your hand on the top of the animal's head. Many animals will want your other hand touching and comforting them under their chin, on the side of their neck, or even on their backbone.

Draw your hand from the crown chakra down the back of its neck, feeling for tension. Settle in between the shoulder blades, breathing deeply.

Next, draw your hands down the backbone to the back of the heart, and hold this spot for a moment.

Collect the third and second chakras downward into the root, and hold for a moment on the base of the tail. You can feel around the animal's hip bones in a gentle massage while you send the Reiki so it does not become nervous about you touching its hindquarters. Gently draw this energy all the way down its tail and flick it outward, just as you did with the third eye.

Take your hands and sandwich the animal's legs one at a time and sweep down and out the feet. Move as fast or slow as the animal wants.

Now, run your hand along the underbelly. Feel for the heart, lungs, and organs. Do not push this on an insecure animal. You can also sandwich the two sides of the pet from the rib cage all the way down to the hind legs.

Animals enjoy a lot of sweeping and flicking. They like having stuck energy flung off and will often yawn, shake, or want to sleep.

You may now go back to any one spot to send more Reiki where you felt a strong pull. Do not trouble yourself trying to sort it out, but do ask the animal's higher self to direct you and give you any information that may be useful.

When you feel you are done, sweep all over the body and out the tail again. You may repeat the third-eye sweep one more time as well.

With animals, it's more useful to stay focused on all the physical sensations you and they are experiencing, rather than trying to focus too much on the chakra centers. Because they are generally more flowing then we are, overfocusing on a single chakra can be counter-effective, causing them to feel stuck rather than helped.

In the case of small animals like hamsters and toads, or animals with strange shapes like hermit crabs or snakes, simply sandwich the whole animal and sweep off the third eye and the tail area three times in a row. If the animal wants your Reiki in a continued flow, it will become very still and just sit there. I once had to ask a toad if she would please get down now!

Most of all, when treating animals, stay open to a deeper state of consciousness in yourself. Try to know less and feel more. Trust the higher self of the animal to be communicating with you, and trust yourself to come from a place of love and well-being.

I find that performing healings on animals not only opens me up in new ways, but they often also teach me things about Reiki that I never knew before. A cat taught me about color Reiki, and a horse showed me how I could encapsulate the colic in it like an oily ooze and pull it out. I have evolved as a healer and human being by not allowing my ego to get involved in the treatments, and to instead dive into deep and open relationships with all beings of nature.

Acknowledgments

It surely takes a village to raise a child, and the same can be said about books. Many thanks to Kelly Sullivan Walden for being my gracious and loving book midwife. Much love to Wendy Capland and the Sheroes; thanks for holding space and believing in me. To Rosanne Romiglio, may we continue to move each other forward with love. Thanks to Jo Spring for some wonderful editing and Kelley Twombly for always having my back. Gratitude to the wonderful team at New Harbinger for holding my hand throughout the process with skill and grace.

Many thanks to Rhys Thomas for the lovely foreword and our long friendship. And, a big thank you to my family and friends for always believing in me and putting up with my absences when the writing overtook me.

Most of all, I want to thank my Reiki students for showing me the way and keeping me humble.

References

Andrews, T. 2006. *How to See and Read the Aura*. Woodbury, NM: Llewellyn Publications.

Hay, L. L. 1984. *You Can Heal Your Life*. Carlsbad, CA: Hay House.

Judith, A. 2004. *Eastern Body, Western Mind: Psychology and the Chakra System as a Path to the Self*. Berkeley, CA: Celestial Arts.

Rand, W. L. 1998. *Reiki for a New Millennium*. Harrisonburg, VA: Vision Publications.

Shapiro, D. 2006. *Your Body Speaks Your Mind: Decoding the Emotional, Psychological, and Spiritual Messages that Underlie Illness*. Boulder, CO: Sounds True.

Stein, D. 1995. *Essential Reiki: A Complete Guide to an Ancient Healing Art*. Berkley, CA: Crossing Press.

Stiene, B. and F. Stiene. 2008. *The Reiki Sourcebook*. Rev. ed. Alresford, UK: O Books.

Thomas, R. 2015. *Discover Your Purpose: How to Use the 5 Life Purpose Profiles to Unlock Your Hidden Potential and Live the Life You Were Meant to Live*. New York: Tarcher/Penguin.

Lisa Campion is a psychic counselor and Reiki master teacher with over twenty-five years of experience. She has trained more than one thousand practitioners in the hands-on, energy-healing practice of Reiki, including medical professionals, and has conducted more than fifteen thousand individual sessions in her career. Based near Boston, MA, she specializes in training emerging psychics, empaths, and healers so they can fully step into their gifts—the world needs all the healers it can get!

Foreword writer **Rhys Thomas** is a visionary author, speaker, trainer, and coach in the personal growth and energy medicine field. He is author of *Discover Your Purpose*, founder of the Rhys Thomas Institute of Energy Medicine, and creator of the Rhys Method®—a powerful system of self-discovery, transformation, and healing.

MORE BOOKS for the SPIRITUAL SEEKER

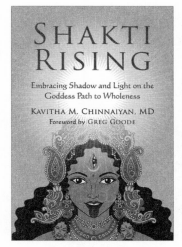
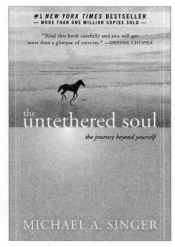
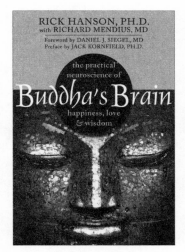
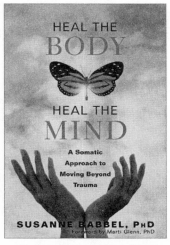
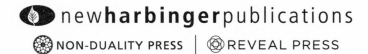

Register your **new harbinger** titles for additional benefits!

When you register your **new harbinger** title—purchased in any format, from any source—you get access to benefits like the following:

- Downloadable accessories like printable worksheets and extra content

- Instructional videos and audio files

- Information about updates, corrections, and new editions

Not every title has accessories, but we're adding new material all the time.

Access free accessories in 3 easy steps:

1. Sign in at NewHarbinger.com (or **register** to create an account).

2. Click on **register a book**. Search for your title and click the **register** button when it appears.

3. Click on the **book cover or title** to go to its details page. Click on **accessories** to view and access files.

That's all there is to it!

If you need help, visit:

NewHarbinger.com/accessories

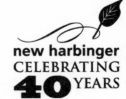